Treatment of the Seriously Ill Psychiatric Patient

Treatment of the Seriously Ill Psychiatric Patient

Edited by
Alexander Gralnick, M.D.

Medical Director, High Point Hospital
Associate Clinical Professor of Psychiatry,
New York Medical College

The Gralnick Foundation
Port Chester/Rye Brook, New York

Published by
THE GRALNICK FOUNDATION
Upper King Street
Port Chester/Rye Brook, N.Y. 10573

Library of Congress Catalog Card No. 83-6071

MANUFACTURED IN THE UNITED STATES OF AMERICA

Dedicated to

Maurice Greenhill, M.D.,

and

Silvano Arieti, M.D.,

eminent psychiatrists and former Chairmen of the Board of Governors of High Point Hospital, whose untimely deaths in 1981 were a great loss to psychiatry.

Preface

In psychiatry, as in medicine generally, there are some patients who are more difficult to treat than others. Despite our best and most honest intentions, the state of our expertise and our intensive efforts often do not seem to be enough. We then speak of these patients as "the seriously ill" and recognize that we have very much to learn about their treatment.

That is why on March 4, 1979, the Albert Einstein College of Medicine and High Point Hospital of Port Chester, New York, jointly sponsored an all-day symposium in New York City to educate mental health professionals on the treatment of the seriously ill psychiatric patient. Experts in the fields of child and adolescent psychotherapy, the psychotherapy of depression, and treatment of borderline and schizophrenic patients were called upon to contribute their knowledge. The present volume represents the proceedings of this symposium.

One of the main functions of the Gralnick Foundation has been the fostering of professional education, and its board of trustees is now happy to support this publication. The spadework in gathering the speakers was done by Dr. Maurice Greenhill, Professor of Psychiatry at Albert Einstein College of Medicine and Chairman of the Board of Governors of High

Point Hospital until his death in 1981. The administrative work for the symposium was done by the Department of Continuing Education at Albert Einstein. It is gratifying that the close working relationship between High Point Hospital and Albert Einstein College proves rewarding and beneficial to the profession at large.

ALEXANDER GRALNICK, M.D.

Contents

Introduction

The symposium which led to this volume focused more on certain types of patients who present particular problems of management and treatment rather than on too wide a spectrum of them.

In Chapter 1, James E. Groves discusses the problems inherent in the care of the exceptionally dependent patient, choosing perhaps unfortunately the term "the hateful patient." While these patients do tend to mobilize extraordinarily negative feelings in care givers, and while his choice of a term is in some ways accurately reflective of the negative countertransference, it is important to realize that it is not really the patients who are hateful but rather the behaviors which evoke the countertransference feelings. Dr. Groves prefers to say that the patients are hateful because he believes this general mode of conceptualization can be useful to the care giver in dealing with these difficult borderline individuals. The reader must judge independently whether it is necessary to so label the patient or if one can still utilize the author's insights without the label.

In Chapter 2, Jules R. Bemporad focuses on the borderline child. Interestingly, most of the chapters focus on borderline character structure, which is becoming an increasingly prevalent clinical problem. Dr. Bemporad correctly states that some of these children also suffer from mild neurologic difficulties. The combination of neurologic deficit with the vicissitudes of psychological growth and development can combine to make particularly difficult treatment problems. Bemporad deals with a number of the technical problems involved in the management and treatment of these seriously disturbed children. He correctly notes the necessity for long-term and continuing treatment if the final outcome is to be successful.

Silvano Arieti, who was so well-known for his contributions to the literature on schizophrenia, had a long interest in the problems of severe depression. As was so often the case during his long and productive life, Dr. Arieti argues in Chapter 3 for balance in our understanding of the etiology and treatment of depression. He does not deny or disparage the value of medication, but merely insists upon the importance of psychological factors as well. It is interesting to realize that many pharmacologists are increasingly becoming aware of the importance of psychotherapeutic treatment as part of the overall management of the severe depressive disorders. Very often these patients live in psychological environments which are likely to contribute to relapse, and if they do not adequately change their social networks and supports, they are at increased risk for recurrence. This is one of Dr. Arieti's last works to be published before his untimely death. His voice of reason and balance will be sorely missed.

Adolescence is a complicated phase of human development. In Chapter 4, Derek H. Miller focuses on those adolescents who fall in the midrange of disturbance between moderate and intractable. He points out that many of these youngsters do not have adequate social supports during the period of adolescence, which contributes to their difficulties. He makes a number of useful points which are of interest to those who treat the adolescent patient.

In the next chapter Gerald J. Sarwer-Foner deals with some

of the problems of the intractable borderline patient. He uses the term to refer to a character disorder which in certain cases is treatable and in other cases is not treatable. He deals with the factors which constitute such a borderline personality organization and the issues which tend to make certain of these patients untreatable. While it is always difficult to accept the fact that some people are untreatable by our present methods, the reality is that such people do exist and in goodly numbers.

In Chapter 6, I argue that the management of the schizophrenic patient when correctly diagnosed is difficult because they are almost all severely ill. I attempt to identify the patients who are best included within the category of the schizophrenic disorders and discuss the range of treatment methods which have proven to be helpful for at least some of these people. Despite the enthusiasm for pharmacotherapy in the schizophrenias, experience suggests that psychotherapeutic interventions are not yet passé.

The vast majority of patients who are seeking psychiatric treatment today fall into the category of the seriously ill. They are considered to be seriously ill because they are not rapidly responsive to the treatment methods available. This is perhaps a misuse of the term "seriously ill" but it does reflect an operational usage which has value. There is a striking consistency of borderline personality features which cuts across diagnostic categories and tends to characterize the more difficult treatment problems. While the difficult to treat patients are not restricted exclusively to the borderline personality organization, this disorder is quite well represented. This volume offers some assistance to the clinician in thinking through the issues of dynamic management and treatment without excluding the utility of pharmacologic intervention.

ROBERT CANCRO, M.D.

Contributors

SILVANO ARIETI, M.D.
Clinical Professor of Psychiatry, New York Medical College, New York

JULES R. BEMPORAD, M.D.
Director of Children's Services, Associate Professor of Psychiatry, Massachusetts Mental Health Center, Harvard Medical School, Boston, Massachusetts

ROBERT CANCRO, M.D.
Professor and Chairman, Department of Psychiatry, New York University Medical Center, New York City, New York

JAMES E. GROVES, M.D.
Clinical Instructor in Psychiatry, Harvard Medical School, Boston, Massachusetts

DEREK H. MILLER, M.D.
Professor of Psychiatry, Northwestern University School of Medicine, Chicago, Illinois

GERALD J. SARWER-FONER, M.D.
Professor and Chairman, Department of Psychiatry, University of Ottawa School of Medicine; Director, Department of Psychiatry, Ottawa General Hospital, Ottawa, Ontario, Canada

Treatment of the Seriously Ill Psychiatric Patient

Chapter 1

Taking Care of the Hateful Patient

James E. Groves, M.D.

I want to discuss the subject I have called "Taking Care of the Hateful Patient." My paper of that name was specifically directed to a readership outside of the mental health field. It was aimed at helping the nonpsychiatric physician, the surgeon, the medical student, the dentist, or any care giver to deal more usefully with the difficult, the obnoxious, the intractable, the threatening patient.

Psychiatrists, psychologists, psychiatric nurses, and social workers who have read the paper of course recognize that I am talking about the pathologically dependent patient, whom I am calling by a different name. Hateful patients are generally patients with character disorders, or so-called borderline patients who present problems to the general hospital or in the offices and clinics of those care givers not dealing primarily with mental health.

My talk today will consist of three parts. First I am going to tell you how the paper came to be written; next I will summarize the paper; and finally I will discuss how I, as a medical-psychiatric consultant, understand and utilize the hateful patient concept in liaison psychiatry.

The paper began one day in November of 1976 when I was

just one and one half years out of my psychiatric residency and into my new office, where I had a part-time practice in general psychiatry. The phone rang and the toneless voice of the mother of a psychotherapy patient of mine told me that my patient had killed herself. She hanged herself, and to her dress she had pinned a note thanking me for my efforts over the past year. I hung up the phone and when the numbness wore off, I started to feel troubled. I reviewed the treatment of this patient, asking myself what I had done wrong, what I had missed, and how I had erred. Nothing immediately materialized.

The patient had been in treatment with half a dozen psychotherapists from the time she was thirteen up to when she died under my care, which was just after her twenty-first birthday. At fifteen she was a heroin addict, and by sixteen she had become a full-time prostitute to support her habit. At nineteen, she developed a raging pelvic inflammatory disease, and eventually she had a total hysterectomy. It was at this time she came into psychiatric treatment with me.

From the outset she clung to me for dear life. She was an almost mute, timid little thing, a waif, who seemed to convey by every nuance and every gesture that I, and only I, had the special power to save her. I was stirred, flattered and felt important. Eventually my feelings of power and specialness began to tarnish a bit as she inundated me with requests for help, for attention, for nurture, for anything and everything I could provide; and eventually, of course, no day was free of her.

She seemed to be able to follow me anywhere by telephone. It eventually got to the point of her having me paged while I was on a beach in Bermuda. Needless to say, at the very next opportunity, I told her in no uncertain terms that unless she confined our work to her therapy hours and an allowance of two emergency phone calls per week, our relationship would have to be terminated. At this juncture she appeared shaken. She understood. And she complied.

Over the next month she seemed to get a little better. She

actually got a job as a cocktail waitress, and she stuck with it. She took a course in modern dance, and she started telling me in her treatment hours what her life had actually been like—a poor little rich girl with frantic, helpless parents. She had an inventory of immense suffering. As she told me her story, she seemed to firm up, to become less wilted, less beaten and then to become rigid. It was almost as if she were writing a novel and had decided that she would like her protagonist.

Unfortunately, along with this new picture of herself, she began to develop a privileged attitude, an arrogant sense that only she had suffered, only she had any worth, and that none of my other patients existed. I didn't really exist. Only she existed.

One morning she stalked into my office and announced that she had stayed up the whole night making a list of every bad thing that had ever happened to her. She produced six typewritten pages, which she threw on my desk. She flung herself into a chair and broke a branch off a nearby plant, a Swedish ivy that I had carefully nurtured from a sprig, and which was the centerpiece, I thought, of my newly decorated office.

"Listen shitball," she said to me, "I got it all on paper. I have totalled it up in black and white. I figure I am the most desperate patient you ever saw in your whole, miserable, snob existence. I am entitled to anything you can give me. You are rich. I suffered. You didn't. Now you are going to pay."

All I could think of was several thousand dollars worth of loans still outstanding to medical school, the Swedish ivy she had desecrated, the beach in Bermuda, and for some perverse reason I also remembered Thomas Sydenham, who wrote in the seventeenth century, doubtless about such patients: "All is caprice. They love without measure those whom they will soon hate without reason." I wondered was it Mark Twain's axiom that no good deed goes unpunished. And I thought of the ivy. Then very quietly at first, but with increasing firmness, I politely took her apart.

I summarized her life as a continual disaster. I gently, but with great interior relish, reminded her that her chances of easily getting another therapist, when she was so notorious in town, were sparse. And I told her that her suffering was not worth the paper that it was written on—that it was paper, play money, Monopoly money, which in the real world wouldn't even buy a cup of coffee. I expatiated on the nature of what is earned and what is not, about what one is entitled to and what one is not, and she left the office pale and quiet.

Following this interview, she underwent a metamorphosis into her third incarnation. She decided that, indeed, psychiatry is a branch of medicine, and that being so, she would become a patient. She went to the library and read at length on diabetes and Sjogren's syndrome and several other diseases. Now, whatever might have been said of her, it would have to be conceded that she had been a good medical patient. Unlike most patients, I think, who have a character disorder and a concurrent medical problem, she had been very cooperative with her several physicians. She took her various medications for the Sjogren's and her eyedrops. She managed her diabetes very well, with the aid of a delightful, grandfatherly internist who knew just how to work with her. She underwent various checkups and diagnostic procedures stoically and with minimal fuss, but things changed after this interview. She went into ketoacidosis three times. She raised holy hell in the surgical clinics. She developed symptoms I hadn't ever heard of—symptoms which a bright, young resident said were pathognomonic of various dread diseases. They called me out to ask me how I could have missed Pemberton's sign, Musset's sign and, of course, Seidel's sign. People from all over town were calling me up. I felt I was becoming known at last. The coup de grace, however, occurred when she took herself to a psychiatrist who was senior to me, and whose office was just across the street. The psychiatrist called me up with, as he put it, the results of his consultation. The patient, he noted, had a family history of depressive disorders, alcoholism, weight loss. She ruminated, she wrung her hands, she had sustained periods of hyperactivity, talkativeness, irritability, expansiveness. She had early morning awakening. As I listened to his voice droning tonelessly on I knew what was coming.

Did I know about manic depressive illness? Had I ever heard of tricyclic antidepressants? Was I perhaps familiar with lithium carbonate? If not, my colleague offered helpfully that he would be willing to follow her medication, while I would be free to confine myself to what I was best able to do, ostensibly nothing. The following week, resigned, I put her on lithium, and the week after that when she had adequate serum levels, I started her on a tricyclic. As I placed the prescription in her hand, I said hopefully, I said prayerfully, that I felt the medication would make her feel better fast.

When she returned the following week, she had a host of new symptoms of schizophrenia, and she mentioned that she had discontinued her psychotropic medications. I noted that there was a paradox here. She was discontinuing her medication precisely at a time when she was becoming more symptomatic. She didn't reply. She paused. She went ahead and talked about her symptoms for the rest of the hour. She got up to go and she turned at the threshold, an afterthought, and said, "Tell me this. Is there an antidepressant that doesn't work so damn fast?"

I'll not dwell much on her fourth incarnation. It contains elements of the first three: the clinging and the phone calls, the entitlement and the demandingness, the myriad of new symptoms that resisted any and all treatment. I felt drained. I felt strangled, on guard, ready to attack her entitlement. I felt depressed and devalued as a physician.

She became increasingly depressed and covertly suicidal. She began to throw herself in harm's way. This fourth phase appeared to be a reckless skating along the edge of life, a kind of tightrope act, Russian roulette. She returned to her heroin habits. She began to hang around with really creepy people. She got herself beaten up. She slept anywhere and sometimes would wake up to discover herself in strange surroundings, not knowing how she got there. Yet, she repeatedly denied that she was trying to die.

Of my countertransference feelings, suffice it to say that I began to have recurrent dreams in which I was told that she died. Wonderful dreams; lovely technicolor dreams; lovely, vivid, serene landscapes. Dreams in which a marvelous sense of peace and relief and freedom supervened.

One of the things that happens, I think, when a patient suicides, is that you have to talk about it. You talk with your spouse at first perhaps, or with a trusted supervisor, and then with your colleagues. People commiserate with you and tell you similar stories. As it happened many of my friends were surgeons, dentists and so on, and the anecdotes I was getting back were very familiar. They all had a few patients that they too dreaded, patients that made them feel drained and empty, patients they wanted to tell off, and patients that never got well or continued to develop new symptoms to replace the old ones. A couple of surgeons told me, in strictest confidence, that they too had patients that they wished would die and get it over with—the alcoholic, the race car driver who constantly got himself into automobile accidents and just barely pulled through each time. Everybody had patients who flouted the regimen and seemed to try to die.

By Christmas I was less troubled by this patient's suicide than the month before. I did a lot of inpatient medical and surgical consultations on the ward and I consulted a screening clinic. I buried myself in my work. Early in January of the next year I wrote the first draft of this paper.

In the following months I showed it around and I read about the difficult patient. But except for Winnicott's article, I didn't really find much that described what I had experienced or what my colleagues had told me about their experiences with such patients.

Eventually, I decided to submit the paper, but I still had no title for it. "The Difficult Patient," "The Exasperating Patient," "The Dependent Patient"—I didn't know what to call it. The emotions I had written about were certainly hateful feelings, but I didn't feel that I could call it that. Patients could be all kinds of things, but certainly not hateful. It didn't seem to be the sort of thing that you said, and worse yet, the paper didn't seem quite complete, as if something were lacking.

During this struggle about the title, the very last thing in the world that I wanted to happen, happened. The dead girl's mother sent me a letter and a package. The letter said that the package contained the dead girl's diary. The mother had found this secret diary in an old suitcase, and she thought that perhaps I would like to have it. I will read you, in its entirety, the entry from September 16, 1976.

"Friday. Dr. G. I wonder where you are tonight. It was a pretty horrible session yesterday, huh. I am sinking fast aren't I. I wish I would hurry up and get it over with. I hate myself. I really do. I wonder what you are doing tonight, and with who you are doing it. I wonder if you have given up. I certainly have. Maybe I will hang on until I am 21. I wonder what it feels like to be grownup. Then I'll know, ha ha. I will tell you this one thing though, Dr. G. I bet I was the most hateful patient you ever had."

Now, hateful patients are not those patients with whom the physician has an ordinary personality clash. They are those occasional patients that non-psychiatrists dread. The dependency of such patients leads to behaviors that group them into four stereotypes: *dependent clingers*, *entitled demanders*, *manipulative help-rejectors*, and *self-destructive deniers*.

Dependent clingers attach themselves to their doctors in search of an inexhaustible source of emotional support, as if the medical relationship can cure all ills and provide complete happiness. They come on as helpless and often naive.

Entitled demanders search for those same emotional supplies but use controlling and punishing behaviors in an attempt to get the doctor to supply them. They display entitlement: a haughty, arrogant attitude of innate deservedness; a privileged attitude, usually unjustified, that they are better than other people, that they have earned any- and everything they see. This entitled attitude is backed up by covert or overt threats of revenge. These demanders, like clingers, are searching for a permanent care-giving relationship. It is just that they do it differently.

Manipulative help-rejectors utilize a third stratagem. They use noncompliance with a medical regimen or hypochondriasis or symptom substitution in an effort to maintain the support they receive in the sick role. They display a smug attitude at times that nothing will help really, but the doctor nonetheless feels obliged to perform miracles.

The fourth category, the self-destructive deniers, are profoundly dependent individuals too, but they seem to have given up hope of ever getting their needs met. They don't listen. They appear oblivious to the dangers of their self-destructiveness. They seem to find their main pleasure in defeating any attempt to help them, and they no longer seem to care whether they live or die.

The type of negative emotion the doctor experiences in response to these four stereotypes of patients is like a laboratory test. If the doctor experiences suffocation and a feeling of aversion toward the patient, the patient is likely to be a clinger. If the doctor is at first afraid of the patient and then begins to feel the urge to counterattack that repulsive sense of innate deservedness, the patient is probably an entitled demander. If the doctor feels depressed and de-skilled at the patient's continued and deliberate failure to comply and respond to treatment, the patient may well be a manipulative help-rejector. If the doctor begins to feel malice toward the patient and eventually begins to wish secretly that the patient would die and get it over with, the patient is probably the self-destructive denier who may embody the chronic and unconscious version of what in its acute conscious form is called suicide.

The prognosis for cure of each of these states or syndromes

or stereotypes by the primary nonpsychiatric physician is poor. The ongoing medical treatment consists of palliative maneuvers by the physician.

Clingers need to be identified early by means of the feelings of aversion they create, and to be told gently and firmly, but as explicitly as possible, that the doctor is going to set limits on the duration and number of visits and, therefore, implicitly on the depth of intimacy of their relationship. These limits on the clingers' expectations for an intense doctor–patient relationship are set so that the patients don't feel rejected, or collapse in despair when disappointments occur, as they inevitably do in any relationship.

Demanders can be identified as entitled by the doctor's wish to devalue them. They need to have their feelings of total deservedness rechanneled into a partnership that acknowledges their entitlement not to unrealistic demands, but to good medical care. While the doctor shouldn't attack the patient's wish for the restoration of what is essentially the parent–child relationship rather than the doctor–patient relationship, the doctor explicitly reassures the patient that there is a real relationship, and that the patient does have rights: the right to the very best possible medical care that can be provided.

Help-rejectors need to learn that losing the symptom does not mean losing the doctor. They manipulate the relationship by staying symptomatic, and yet they reject whatever help is offered. This paradox is a maladapted solution to the need–fear dilemma and it illustrates that they simultaneously crave intimacy, and yet have a terrible fear of that same intimacy.

To resolve this Catch-22, the physician may have to resort to a countermaneuver that consists of finding the middle ground between the patient's wish to fuse and the patient's fear of being gobbled up. The physician begins by recognizing his or her own feelings of pessimism, and then states honestly that the treatment is not a panacea. Thus, even if improvements in the patient's condition do occur, the medical relationship will still need to be maintained over time, but at regular intervals determined by the physician, not by the patient's manipulation through symptoms.

Self-destructive deniers need to be distinguished from healthy deniers, who utilize denial generally in service of emotional stability, not as a manifestation of indifference to being alive. Healthy deniers usually don't stir up malice. Self-destructive deniers are altogether different. They are best managed in the context of the doctor realizing that without shame, or without self-blame, that such patients do evoke hate, and they do confound the expertise of even the most ideal care giver. Realizing that he or she is doing the best any doctor could helps the physician to combat the urge to abandon the patient, to act with perseverence and compassion, just as one would with any other patient with a terminal illness.

I want to use the final third of my talk to tell you about how I use the hateful patient concept in my work with the physician-consultee. As you now know, hateful patients are patients whose ego functions are at the borderline level, or patients who are at the borderline level and who happen to appear in the medical-surgical context. Their object relations are principally transitional.

For me what stands out about the borderline patient who becomes the hateful patient by means of his or her entry into the medical care system, is that such patients greatly use entitlement and manipulativeness as defenses, and habitually use splitting and projective identification. Of the many things that one could watch for in borderline phenomenology on the medical-surgical ward, the most important things to look for are entitlement, manipulativeness, defensive splitting and projective identification. That is because of their devastating impact on the physician-consultee's self-esteem.

Entitlement is the emotionally deprived individual's attempt to collect *now* what he ought to have gotten back *then*. Babies really are entitled to be babied; otherwise they wouldn't survive. But adults who wish to collect on those same promises of care giving we call entitled.

What happens in the hospital or doctor's office is that the dependent individual attempts to wrest from the doctor–patient relationship that which he or she didn't get from the mother–child relationship. Of course this doesn't work. But if one tries to tell entitled individuals the facts of life they usually only become more entitled. Or worse, they panic; they regress to even more primitive levels. In other words, the entitlement may act as a defense to the actions of borderline patients. It is a bad defense, an inefficient defense that only makes things worse at times, but it is the best defense that they have available at that particular moment.

Thus, with the entitled patient, time and again we observe the physician-consultee getting tired, drained and frightened, and finally counterattacking the patient's entitlement head on. What this is, is the physician telling the patient that the medical relationship isn't the mother–child relationship. But entitlement is the borderline patient's religion to gainsay; it is a kind of blasphemy, a kind of stripping away of that which is felt by the patient to give life its meaning, and to give adversity its cure. It is a primitive, wanton belief that one *deserves*.

Such an attitude may enrage the physician, especially if his or her own defenses are shaky and if there is a regression on the doctor's part towards his or her own entitlement as a defense. What I, as a consultant, try to do in the medical-surgical context is to get the consultee not to attack the defensive entitlement of the patient, but rather to attempt to substitute the medical relationship itself as a defense against the patient's fear of abandonment.

Manipulativeness has a defensive function for the patient too, similar to that of entitlement. For instance, as I have said, help-rejecting is the patient's maladaptive compromise solution to the need–fear dilemma. Again, what I as a consultant try to do is to get the consultee not to attack defensive manipulativeness, but rather to attempt to substitute for it the medical relationship. I counsel the consultee to share a kind of pessimism with the patient by saying to the patient something along the lines of "Well, this you know is a chronic condition, and we may never entirely cure it. We will have to keep on with our relationship." By such tactics, especially by giving the consultee permission to be candid, and to be less than perfect, the consultant takes a lot of pressure out of the relationship because the care giver has something to do. He or she can substitute the relationship for the manipulativeness.

You are very familiar with how borderline patients use splitting as a defense, and of course they do so dramatically in the medical context. For instance, they frequently see one care giver as omnipotent and omniscient, while at the same time they devalue and denigrate another. They utilize an idealizing transference to protect themselves, not only from the illness, but also from their own projected envy and rage.

I have used the term "clinger" to denominate the borderline's using the physician as a transitional object. As you and I know, the clinger's adoration is not object love. It is like getting a letter in the mail which says "I love you, I love you, I love you," and then realizing the letter is addressed to "occupant." But the doctor who doesn't recognize that the adulation that he or she is getting from the clinger is marked "occupant" is prone to reciprocate as if it were object love, and thus to overstimulate the patient. It is not good, of course, to tear away the patient's idealization altogether since it serves a good defensive function; but for those with unfillable emptiness, there is no such thing as "enough." The care giver who attempts to supply "enough" will end up giving too much, overstimulating the patient, exhausting the doctor's capacity to care, and eventually abandoning the patient.

The other half of the splitting mechanism is seen when the patient uses projective identification to dump his or her own pathology or pathologic content onto the physician, particularly envy and rage. As you know, projective identification differs from mere projection in several respects. In projection, a disowned affect or impulse is conferred upon the object. In projective identification, not only the affect or impulse is conferred, but along with it a whole personality trait or disposition is projected. Moreover, in projective identification, the person projecting holds on to part of the affect, and also reacts to that which is projected. In other words, projective identification is the glue for a pathologic bond.

In projective identification, there is an almost uncanny tendency for the victim or object of the projection to begin to enact and eventually to validate the projection. This phenomenon is so important in consultations involving the hateful patient that I want to give you an example.

Several weeks ago, I was called by a colleague to consult about some patient on the oncology floor. He and I were talking about it afterwards in the hall when coincidentally another one of his patients accosted my colleague. So I happened to be right on the scene when the projective identification was taking place.

Now, I had known my oncologist friend for years as a kind, stable man, the son of a family of physicians that stretched back three generations. He was a person who always had a need to serve, to be helpful to people, almost to excess, and he was, in my view, and is a generous, nonauthoritarian, flexible, empathic person. The patient, I found out later, was a fifty-year-old fundamentalist preacher, a man with leukemia in good remission; a volatile, plethoric man, whose intolerance was matched only by his ignorance. Despite a good result from years of chemotherapy, he devalued doctors, savagely calling them "quacks and ungodly meddlers who work more against, than with, the holy spirit." He was envious of physicians and he was obviously jealous of what he saw as unearned, unwarranted social status and financial security. He saw physicians as a secretive closed guild, incestuous and corrupt, plotting to exclude legitimate competition. At the time of this encounter he had already, unknown to us, signed out against medical advice in the presence of his wife, the hospital lawyer and his internist. Now remember that the oncologist and I didn't know this; we were totally unaware of this.

What happened was that the patient stalked up to my friend

and loudly stated that he was leaving the hospital to begin a course of Laetrile treatment. Furthermore, he shouted, his act not only represented his determination to survive but symbolized his protest against the medical establishment and its unfair monopoly.

My friend gently remonstrated with this patient and urged him to reconsider. He expressed respect for the patient's viewpoint but disagreement with it, and in general he undertook to dissuade this patient from leaving the hospital. I was standing there and I must confess I detested this patient. I saw him as a mouth-breathing bigot and I just couldn't think of enough bad things to do to him. After a few minutes, I tuned in again and I was amazed to note a change in my friend and colleague.

As they talked, the doctor became peevish, defensive and arrogant and got red in the face. He stammered and avoided eye contact. He contradicted himself. He began to misrepresent the actual situation, and eventually he fell to telling outright lies. He resorted to counterthreats. He utilized ad hominem arguments and he started to devalue the patient. In short, my friend got into an absolute swivet over the loss of this patient. The patient had gotten him to enact the projection, to become what the patient expected, to become what the patient wished and decreed.

I can't emphasize enough that the consultee with the hateful patient is having a drastic, shocking burden placed on his or her self-esteem. And when the patient inflicts a narcissistic injury on the doctor, the doctor attacks those very defenses that the patient needs for survival during the vicissitudes of a medical or surgical illness.

In the example of my psychotherapy patient, when her idealization crumbled, devaluation followed; and when her defensive entitlement was stripped away, the defensive, hypochondriacal, manipulative help-rejecting was substituted. Eventually, when she had no defenses and no relationship, she died.

It is precisely this pathological interaction between the

dependent and depressed patient and the narcissistically injured doctor that the hateful patient concept is designed to remedy. When I am asked to consult in the medical or surgical context, I use the stereotypes clinger, demander, help-rejector and self-destructive denier to symbolize and embody how borderline patients behave and how they may most easily be helped in the short run. This labelling maneuver is supportive of the physician-consultee and helps restore intellectual defenses against the loss of self-esteem by the doctor who is taking care of the hateful patient.

The clinger, for instance, is a metaphor for the idealizing transference. By so labelling the patient, you help the consultee resist overstimulating the patient in the early part of the relationship and abandoning the patient in the later part. All that glitters is not gold, and the psychiatric consultant's teaching provides the real gold of knowledge about dependent patients to help protect the physician-consultee against the fool's gold of primitive idealizing transference love and his or her reaction to it.

The demander is a metaphor for the attitudes of envy and entitlement that the patient has toward the doctor. By explaining to the doctor how entitled demanders are, the consultant illustrates the defensive nature of entitlement and the way to work with it, rather than against it. Also, it protects the care giver's self-esteem so that he or she is more easily able to resist the patient's projective identifications. In other words, by using the term "demander" to support and teach the doctor, you shore up his or her self-esteem so that there is a lessened tendency for pathologic interpsychic contents to get dumped onto the doctor.

The term "help-rejector" similarly supports and teaches the physician and immunizes him or her from the punitive attacks by the presumptuous, sadistic superego for not curing the patient. This idea about the doctor's superego is so important that I want to end the talk on that subject.

I don't think that an individual would go into a career as

punishing as medicine if he or she didn't have either an unrealistically exalted ego-ideal or an unrealistically stern superego, or both. When you are an intern, asleep at 4 A.M., and you are awakened to admit an alcoholic who is bleeding from both ends, I don't think you can get up unless there is an angelic ego-ideal saying "Darling, you are wonderful. Get up and save him," and a hellish superego saying "You jerk, if you don't get up, I am going to kick your ass out of that bed." Later on, mellowing usually occurs and self-esteem firms up. Ego-ideal becomes calm. Realistic superego largely loses its sadism and ego generally prevails, but hateful patients are always able to stir up primitive conflicts of self-worth in the doctor.

I think that projective identification by the patient is acted out only when there is some empty space in the doctor's self-esteem. The patient cannot dump pathologic interpsychic contents onto the physician and have him or her own them, unless there is some lacuna in the physician's self-esteem. But firstly, primitive patients are experts at finding these lacunae in the doctor. Secondly, all of us have such holes in our self-esteem. Thirdly, punitive superego enlarges these lacunae. Therefore, when the psychiatric consultant supports the physician's ego, or interposes between physician and punitive superego, the physician's tendency to interject pathologic interpsychic contents from the patient is lessened or stopped altogether.

It is for this reason that I devised the stereotype of the self-destructive denier. The self-destructive denier concept is intended to illustrate to the physician how borderline patients generate trouble and to absolve the physician from blame for this trouble—to get him or her out from under the tremendously punitive superego.

Since I think that most physicians have an obsessive, omnipotent streak, I think they feel partly responsible for everything that occurs. And certain acts of the borderline patient make the physician yearn for the patient to die and get it over with, which in turn stirs up guilt, shame and depression in the consultee. When the consultant discerns this unbidden, unwanted wish in the physician-consultee and correctly replaces this wish back into the patient, he or she stabilizes the care giver's beleaguered ego, diminishes punitive superego, plugs ego lacunae, lessens projective identification by the patient onto the doctor, and generally restores a less conflicted doctor–patient relationship.

To the extent that the consultant can use the self-destructive denier concept specifically and the hateful patient concept generally to protect the physician-consultee's self-esteem, the consultant can resist the borderline patient's projective identifications. When this occurs, the physician is freer not to act hatefully toward the hateful patient.

Chapter 2

The Seriously Disturbed Child

Jules R. Bemporad, M.D.

Before we can adequately discuss the treatment of the seriously disturbed child, we have to be able to propose certain diagnostic criteria by which to identify such a child. While agreed upon measures of severity of illness may not present a problem in the evaluation of adults, unfortunately this is not the case in child psychiatry. The major obstacle to accurate diagnostic assessment in childhood psychiatric illness is that, in contrast to adults, children are unfinished, rapidly changing individuals. What is fully differentiated and stable in the adult is manifested in a global and transient manner by the child.

If an adult presents with a confusion of fantasy and reality, together with peculiar usage of thought and extremes of affect, we rightly suspect an underlying schizophrenic disorder. However, at times the younger child normally fuses fantasy and reality, and older children may demonstrate idiosyncratic thought patterns, as well as a lability of affect. Thus much of what is classified as pathological in the adult is part of the repertoire of normal children. Similarly, symptoms appear and disappear spontaneously in children in the course of development. The causes of such symptoms may be difficulty mastering a new developmental task, adjustment to environmental changes, or even the normal growth of cognitive abilities which make the child aware of new conflicts which he cannot as yet adequately resolve. The child may realize more than he can understand and react to this state of tension with transient symptoms. Familiar examples of these symptoms complexes are the stranger anxiety of the infant, the seemingly irrational fears of the preschooler, and the obsessional behavior of the latency age child. Therefore, symptoms, taken in isolation, are not much help in gauging the severity of psychopathology in children.

The two other indices which are often useful in assessing the severity of disturbance in the adult, namely the degree of subjective discomfort and the impairment of functioning, are equally unreliable in the child. Actually, children may suffer more over trivial disappointments in reality than as a result of malignant pathological inner forces. Often, some symptoms such as encopresis or enuresis are more disturbing to the parent than to the child. Finally, the level of functioning in most children is so inconsistent and responsive to external events that stability of functioning is a mythical ideal.

In view of these impediments to adequate assessment, how can the practitioner reliably determine the degree of severity of illness in any child patient? Some clinicians appear to have given up the attempt to formulate a diagnosis on the basis of the underlying personality and, instead, simply record the presenting symptoms without really delving deeper into their possible meanings or causes. I believe this view is reflected in the DSM-II which, while listing diagnoses which can be easily identified and tabulated, does not tell us much about what is going on in the child. As a result, most clinicians use the catchall label of "adjustment reaction of childhood" to apply to a plethora of diverse conditions.

In a radically different manner, Anna Freud and her colleagues (1965) have pursued the problem of assessment and have come up with a rather accurate and heuristic diagnostic schema that goes beyond superficial symptoms to a deeper level of conceptualization. The key to Freud's system is to always think of the child as a developing being and to conceive of health as the normal progression of development. Pathology, therefore, can be seen as the type and extent of developmental stasis or deviation, regardless of symptoms, suffering or momentary interference of functioning. These latter manifestations become important when they either result from a chronic blockage of the developmental process or themselves impede that very process. Let me quote Anna Freud here: "Play, freedom of fantasy life, school performance, stability of object relations, social adaptation have, all of them, been suggested in turn as vital aspects. Nevertheless, not one of them can qualify as being on a par with the adult's two vital functions: his capacity to lead a normal love and sex life and his capacity to work . . . there is only one factor in childhood, the impairment of which can be considered of sufficient importance in this respect, namely, the child's capacity to move forward in progressive steps until maturation, development in all areas of the personality, and adaptation to the social community have been completed. Mental upsets can be taken as a matter of course so long as these vital processes are left intact. They have to be taken seriously as soon as development itself is affected, whether slowed up, reversed, or brought to a standstill altogether (Freud, 1965, p. 123). Therefore, in assessing the severity of psychopathology, the clinician must attempt to determine the areas in which the developmental process has been blocked or has subsequently deviated from the norm, the extent of this arrest and the sources which continue to impede progress toward maturity.

Some seriously disturbed children give evidence of having been arrested in development in only one area of functioning, but this area is so crucial that deviant development spreads to other spheres of functioning. A typical example of this situation is the child who has suffered prolonged affective deprivation. If this deprivation is experienced in infancy then a multiplicity of defects can be observed later, since so many other functions, which in the adult are readily separated, are still syncretically fused in the infant. Therefore, failure to receive appropriate stimulation in one crucial area can concurrently affect the growth of other areas of functioning.

If affective deprivation is experienced later, after the functions of the child have differentiated to some extent, one may find a persistence of immature forms of relating to others, without an arrest in other areas of functioning. Cognitive ability, impulse regulation and reality testing progress normally. But since interpersonal relationships are such a vital aspect of psychic life, the intact areas are diverted from productive, autonomous use and are employed in the service of gaining immediate and shallow gratification. This powerful perversion of the intact function toward deviant goals allows us to consider children exhibiting these mechanisms as severely disturbed. This opinion is confirmed by the finding that, without treatment, children with affective deprivation often become adult psychopaths.

An example of such a child was Betty, who presented at age 11 with a history of petty thievery, school truancy and suspected sexual promiscuity. On evaluation, Betty was a peculiar sight to behold: her thin, still girlish body was clothed in tight Levi's, high heels and rather ornate jewelry. Her behavior might be best characterized as a rather poor caricature of Mae West in a 1930's vintage movie. Betty had ceased to apply her superior intelligence to her schoolwork and her considerable talents as an artist, gymnast and dancer had atrophied. She blatantly bragged that she didn't care for anyone, trusted no one and just wanted to have a "good time," whatever that meant.

History revealed that Betty had been a normal, healthy infant born into a stable middle-class family. Her natural mother did not appear to have really desired children but went along with her maternal responsibilities in a duty-bound, if somewhat austere, manner. Betty progressed normally until she was about age three, when her mother began a liaison with another man. At this time, she started neglecting Betty, who gradually began to withdraw into herself. A divorce ensued and following the parents' separation Betty was even more isolated. At age six, Betty was expected to cook her own meals and did not know when her mother would return from work or if she would bring a boyfriend. Betty evolved a fantasy world of her own which she created under the basement stairs. She actually created a home within a home, filled with movie magazines and her own television set. Eventually, when Betty was nine, her father brought charges against his former wife and, after he had remarried, was able to obtain custody of his daughter. When Betty went to live with her father and stepmother, there was an initial honeymoon period. She seemed so sweet and endearing, so grateful for what she was given. However, soon it was perceived that beneath this superficial, ingratiating facade, Betty was stealing, lying and showing very little concern for the welfare of others. This double stance also characterized Betty's behavior at school, where she presented as an innocent, well-meaning child and then did not do her work or cut classes at will.

Betty's parents responded with anger and increasing restrictions and punishments, to which Betty at first secretly and later openly rebelled, until she was constantly at odds with the family, who vacillated between anger and guilt. At this point, Betty expressed a great desire to see her natural mother on a regular basis, which was allowed because the family believed Betty was showing some concern for at least one adult. It was soon learned, however, that Betty wanted to see her mother because the latter would routinely give her money with which Betty would buy forbidden items such as jewelry or cosmetics.

Betty presented as an originally healthy child whose development of interpersonal relationships had been arrested at the stage of the need-fulfilling other, when other people are perceived only for what they can give to one, in a concrete manner typical of the preschooler age of development. Therapy had to aim at creating a type of environment that would allow this arrest to be overcome and for more mature relationships to evolve. The parents were seen frequently in order to explain to them Betty's limitations and to prevent them from expecting too much from her. Betty's stepmother was encouraged to enlist Betty in sharing enjoyable work around the house in a manner that would be appropriate for a much younger child. It was also suggested that material rewards be used for good behavior but that such tangible rewards be gradually replaced by verbal praise. Finally, it was suggested that Betty's accomplishments, in school and in her art work, be fussed over in an effort to get Betty to value herself through her creations and accomplishments. It was repeatedly explained that beneath Betty's either rough or excessively compliant facade was a gaping need for care and consideration.

In the therapy sessions, Betty was accepted without criticism. Interpretations were given in matter-of-fact, reality-oriented terms. It was pointed out that Betty did not have to con people for them to like her. It was also stated that she could gain more satisfaction from playing it straight than by sneaking or cheating. She brought in art work which was highly and justifiably praised and also demonstrated new gymnastic stunts in the office hallway. The therapist did not attempt to become the source or object of love—a role left to the parents—however, a positive attachment was demonstrated when Betty brought in a handmade valentine card.

In short, improvement was sought not on the basis of interpretations or even transference manipulation, but on the basis of a corrective emotional experience which hopefully would take place in Betty's new relationship with her parents. This aim was gradually achieved, with Betty becoming more responsible and responsive. It appeared that development along the path of relationships was progressing and with it a freeing up of cognitive and other talents for more productive use.

This case has been selected because it represents the effect of late maternal deprivation in almost pure culture. Betty's problems were not compounded by poverty, asocial attitudes and intellectual sterility as found in underprivileged children. Therefore the effect of deprivation is more clearly definable and perhaps treatable. However, the other reason for the selection of this case is to show the tenuous nature of the progress that has been so laboriously achieved. Betty continued to do well for two years, until her stepmother decided she wanted her own child. The birth of a new baby proved threatening to Betty and aroused her jealousy, for she perceived it as a betrayal and proof that no one could really love her, that demonstrations of love were false and transient. She ran away from home and when returned was enraged with her parents. They felt they could no longer control her and feared for the safety of the baby. After much soul-searching, it was agreed to send Betty to a residential treatment center, even though she might perceive this as a certain rejection. In this new setting, she rapidly regained her achievements and has done well.

If Betty's course has been difficult as the result of an arrest in one area of development, then what can be said about children who manifest delayed development progress in a number of crucial areas? I am not referring to children with autism or symbiotic psychosis because, although these youngsters are obviously disturbed, we still do not know enough about the nature of the disturbance. Autistic children appear to suffer from an as yet unknown organic lesion, with varying degrees of severity and varying amounts of associated gross brain damage. The treatment for such youngsters is leaning toward cognitive stimulation and social training, much like what is done with retarded children. I am not sure that anyone has been able to correlate long-term improvement and any form of treatment. What I do know is that autistic children do not lend themselves to, nor do they seem to profit from, traditional psychotherapy.

Fortunately, autistic children are rare and symbiotic children are even rarer. On the other hand, there is a large group of children who are frequently seen, who present severe forms of pathology and are amenable to psychotherapeutic intervention. These children have been called pseudoschizophrenic, borderline, atypical, severely neurotic or are said to have severe personality disorders. There does not appear to be an adequate diagnostic label for them, although they present a fairly consistent picture. One of the cardinal features of such children is profound anxiety that cannot be mastered and overwhelms the child without warning. Fred Pine (1974) correctly describes these children as lacking "signal anxiety" so that they cannot ward off the occurrence of a pervasive sense of terror in stressful situations. In this regard, they appear to evidence a picture somewhat similar to that which Goldstein (1939) described in adult, organically damaged patients by his concept of "catastrophic reaction." These children try to avoid this terror by withdrawal and isolation; they really cannot manage a normal social existence since it is fraught with the possibility of this sense of internal disintegration. Frequently, during these episodes of terror, the children may appear psychotic: they may act bizarrely, have temper outbursts, hurt themselves or others. Yet as quickly as they disintegrate, they reintegrate and again come into contact with reality. They are thus quite different from those rare children with prolonged psychotic or schizophrenic episodes who lose contact with reality for long periods of time. It is my impression that this lack of defense and the quality of the anxiety experienced represent an organic impairment, although the nature of such a defect has never been specified. Nevertheless, the global, overwhelming nature of their anxiety attacks suggests a primitive, undifferentiated neurological status in which affects cannot be localized and managed. This early, and possibly organic, arrest creates further blocks to development since these very experiences of terror impede normal growth. In later life this intense anxiety takes the form of severe phobias and obsessions, when these children become cognitively able to muster these feeble defenses. In contrast to neurotic youngsters, their fears or rituals have an eerie, desperate and magical quality that often relates to a dread of annihilation.

Other possibly organic derivatives are these children's concrete thought processes and failure to grasp nuances of language and social interaction, despite high intelligence. For example, one such 11-year-old youngster was helping to welcome guests at a family get-together at his house. A distant uncle whom he had met a few times asked jokingly, "And whose little boy are you?" The child experienced a sense of panic at this remark. He knew that he had met the uncle, yet the uncle did not seem to recognize him. He thought that perhaps people did not know who he was any longer. The boy ran to his room and refused to come out for the rest of the evening, believing that he was no longer the same as he had been, since others no longer knew him.

Anna Freud (1956) reports a similar concrete distortion of language in a young boy who was fascinated by the London railway station called King's Cross. For this child, this was not a name but the image of a king, cross with his subjects, who chops off their heads. Such misinterpretations are not infrequently found in very young children, but in those borderline youngsters they persist well into late latency, although only in limited areas. There is not the overall concreteness or gross distortion as seen in psychotic youngsters. Therefore, these children show arrests of development in their cognitive processes, in the primitiveness of defenses, and in their inability to modulate emotional states.

Finally, borderline children show abnormalities in human relationships. They utilize others to fulfill infantile needs and may literally cling to others indiscriminately. They may use trusted others, such as parents, as auxiliary egos, fearing to venture forth without them. When in extrafamilial surroundings they are usually withdrawn and preoccupied with their own thoughts and fantasies, although they may occasionally make inappropriate requests of others. For example, the boy mentioned above was referred for psychological testing at age 12. He was at first shy and fearful, so the experienced examiner spent some time getting him to relax. As he became less apprehensive, he asked her for a glass of orange juice. It did not seem out of the ordinary to him that a psychologist, in a regular office, should have a supply of juice on hand.

So far I have stressed the inherent weaknesses of the child, almost as if the disorder were solely due to some unfolding neurological or maturational deficit. Although I believe that an organic disability predisposes to the developmental arrest and deviance, every such child that I have seen came from a family that was rife with marital discord, frequent fighting and a general lack of structure and security. It would appear that this chaotic environment magnifies the innate difficulty to grossly pathological proportions. The siblings of such patients also do not escape the effect of their home environment and frequently present with neurotic or delinquent symptomatology. However, their intact organic state appears to protect them from the severity of decompensation seen in the so-called borderline child.

Conversely, I have seen children who present the same forms of organic impairment as can be grossly assessed by neuropsychological testing who manage with their difficulties and lead fairly normal lives. These children have been blessed with a structured, secure and loving home environment. The parents intuitively seem to be empathetically in touch with their child's discomfort and early bewilderment, and so appear to compensate for the innate lack of organization. On the other hand, the youngster who develops borderline type features in latency has not had the benefit of a warm atmosphere to positively balance early feelings of confusion and disorganization. Quite possibly, the eventual outcome is a result of the amount of constitutional vulnerability versus environmental stress, as originally proposed by Freud and more recently suggested by Goldfarb in his studies of childhood schizophrenia (1961).

In order to flesh out this somewhat dry skeleton of clinical symptoms, I would like to present a brief sketch of a borderline child. This 10½-year-old boy, whom I shall call Billy, was referred initially for poor school performance and aggressive outbursts. A year previously, he had had a trial of an analytic type of therapy with a somewhat classical therapist who observed Billy play and made interpretations. Billy refused to continue this treatment after six months, stating that his therapist sometimes ate lunch during the sessions but refused to share his food. I do not know whether this was in fact true, but Billy's perception of the therapy situation showed that he was more concerned with the more immature gratification of eating than with entering into a true therapeutic alliance, aimed at solving his problems. This finding alone would suggest a severe developmental arrest in a 10½-year-old boy.

During the diagnostic interviews, Billy presented as a pudgy boy who appeared much younger than his chronological age. He seemed frightened and rocked in his chair, which pointed to a syncretic overflow of emotion into motoric channels. At first he volunteered very little but after he relaxed with the use of drawings, and, in his case, the offer of cookies, he rapidly explained that he was no good at school, at home or at play. He experienced himself as constantly criticized without knowing why. He complained of teasing from other children and of chronic fighting between his parents, which frightened him. He also described experiences of total loss of control when he became terrified or angry. He told of a sense of overwhelming panic during thunderstorms, when forced to go swimming, or when his parents had a particularly serious argument. His attacks of anger emerged when he was severely teased, when he could not understand his school assignments, when his siblings messed up his room and his things, or when he suffered a major disappointment or frustration. His day to day existence was one of constant apprehension, fearing attack from without or eruption from within. His few moments of security were when he was alone in his room either playing like a five-year-old with toy cars or reading rather advanced fiction. At night he frequently experienced nightmares concerning death or mutilation.

Past history revealed many significant areas of difficulty. The parents had never gotten along. They were both wealthy and spoiled individuals who had difficulty coping with the responsibilities of marriage and child rearing. While consciously trying to be good parents and providers of care, they repeatedly reacted with bitter anger whenever their own desires were thwarted because of the needs of others, including their children.

Billy exacerbated these pre-existing parental problems. He was a difficult infant: he would cry inordinately, he did not rapidly adjust to a feeding and sleeping schedule, and he did not seem to like being held. Developmental milestones were uneven: he seemed to be an alert, intelligent infant, but he did not walk until 18 months of age and did not talk until he was three. This last developmental delay was especially frustrating for Billy, who would get furious and throw tantrums when he could not make his wishes known. When he did begin to speak, he demonstrated a good vocabulary and high verbal ability.

At age four, he was sent to a nursery school without protest. However, at the school he was quiet and did not relate easily. He also frequently climbed up on the teacher's lap to be held, as a younger child might. When he started public school, he seemed to be in his own world and there was some question regarding how much instruction he was absorbing. He surprised his teachers by showing a complete grasp of what he had been taught.

Handwriting was a problem, as were letter reversals and difficulties with organization. In contrast, reading was advanced. At age nine he was seen by a pediatric neurologist, who found evidence of a minimal organic impairment but also correctly noted that, at this time, the preponderance of Billy's problems were psychological.

Throughout his school years, Billy made no friends, was frightened of other children and only peripherally involved himself in classroom activities. At home, he sometimes played with his much younger brothers and their friends or he would remain isolated in his room, repetitively playing the same sequence with toy cars and trucks. In many ways, he put more and more strain on a family that was barely coping. For example, when everyone was supposed to be preparing to go on a family trip, Billy would be found in his room calmly playing with cars, appearing oblivious to the fact that he should be getting himself ready and that he was causing a delay in plans. Actually, it may well have been the added tension to the household preparations for a trip produced that caused Billy to withdraw into himself. The effect for the family, however, was of yet another inconvenience because of Billy's lack of consideration for others.

To sum up, when Billy presented at age 10½, he revealed severe arrests and deviant development in almost all areas of functioning. Neurological aspects of behavior reflected a lack of differentiation; he was overwhelmed by feelings and reacted to affects with total motoric expression. Socially, he was incapable of true mutual play, was awkward in interpersonal situations and could not grasp the nuances of social communication. Cognitively, he fluctuated between high achievement in aesthetic and linguistic ability, while he retained the impressionistic and animistic distortions of a much younger child. Psychodynamically, he had not developed age appropriate defense mechanisms against the anxiety from within and the frustrations from without. Finally, due to his situation and other factors, Billy had not and was currently not making much progress in order to correct these deviations. With a few exceptions, psychological growth remained stagnant, causing a further gap between actual and expected behavior with each passing year.

How, then, is one to supply treatment for a youngster who presents these myriad and overwhelming arrests in the developmental process? Well, it is obviously not easy and not always rewarding. The difficulties presented by borderline children can be divided into the practical and the theoretical. The practical limitations, although not always talked about, are quite considerable. Since these children have difficulties in so many areas of life, one has to coordinate academic placement, after-school activities, and family interactions. There are frequent phone calls and meetings with others who are involved in the child's care and one feels drained by the multiple contacts that have to be coordinated. These children also require almost daily structuring and support so that sessions must be frequent—at least three times a week. They learn from constant emotional exposure and do not easily carry home interpretations that might be put into use between sessions, so that sessions have to become part of their daily activity. Added to this frequency of therapeutic encounters is the length of actual treatment. This can stretch out to six or seven years. This is not only to insure consolidation of change but also because new developmental tasks, especially those of early adolescence, may undo a great deal of what has been achieved.

Finally, there is the problem of the parents. As mentioned, these children may come from chaotic families so that sterling therapeutic work during the sessions can be nullified by the adverse environment at home. Therefore, the parents must be seen frequently and engaged in the therapeutic process. They must be made aware of their child's difficulties and how to cope with these at home. Since many of the parents are disturbed themselves, the sharing of information and collaboration of effort necessitates tact, patience and, primarily, stamina on the part of the therapist.

The theoretical difficulties also relate to the multiple developmental deficits these children present. There is a tendency not to know where to start and to be overwhelmed by the amount of pathology. Reversing the usual metaphor, one has difficulty seeing the trees for the forest. It is sometimes helpful to organize a list of target symptoms, each with its own treatment goal, and not to rely on objectives gradually evolving from the therapeutic process itself. First, the anxiety must be reduced. Again, these children experience a sense of terror that is more overwhelming than in most individuals and this terror comes without warning. It is like an axe that can fall at any time. Later in therapy the child will learn to identify those situations that evoke the anxiety and eventually to deal with them by psychological means, but at the outset external controls are often necessary. I have found that the majority of such children benefit from psychotropic medications during the initial part of therapy. Phenothiazines, despite their dangers, have proven most effective in diminishing anxiety, while the minor tranquilizers offer little benefit. These medications also help in reducing the anger attacks. Ultimately, they make the child less fearful and less aggressive, and thus more acceptable to himself and others. Billy, for example, was started on 30 mg. Mellaril with a considerable alleviation of the depth of his anxiety and a complete abolishment of the loss of control in his temper outbursts. Often it is best to give these medications in one dose at bedtime, for the rapid sedative effects do not interfere with daytime activity but help the child go to sleep, while the tranquilizing effects continue to the following day. A p.r.n. dose can be given if needed during the day. Billy was so relieved by the medication that he liked to carry around a 10 mg. Mellaril tablet with him, "just in case." He never used it but just the idea that he could do something about his anxiety and temper was significantly reassuring. It initiated a sense of control over his painful feelings and troublesome behavior for the first time. Later, another external support was mutually discovered, his bedside radio. Billy utilized the radio almost like a transitional object. It offered him security and he projected upon it magical, soothing qualities. When upset or sad, he would go to his room and listen to his own radio, sometimes with headphones, and shortly he became calmer and more reasonable. Again, he knew that he could depend upon something in his environment to help protect him against his overwhelming feelings. Another weapon in Billy's fight against the engulfing emotional states was his relationship with his therapist. He knew he could call the therapist at almost any time in the evenings and be given a hearing for his problems. In these instances the therapist had to say very little. Just the fact that Billy felt someone was listening to him often sufficed to quiet his fears or anger.

This brings us to the second crucial objective of the initial stages of therapy: formation of a close relationship with the therapist. This aspect of treatment will remain the key therapeutic factor throughout, and without it real change rarely can take place. For it is ultimately only within this dyadic relationship that the child can find the acceptance of a formerly-criticized self, the ability to face his deficits, the resources for change and growth, and the courage to try new forms of relating outside the office. While the therapist serves different functions at different times, he is primarily a bridge to reality. He must learn the internal distortions of the child and eventually replace these with a more correct interpretation of the real world. As with an adult patient who is severely disturbed, the therapist should, at first, accept the distorted representation of reality, but with an eye to later tracing the origins of the delusions and thus correcting them. It would have been pointless to argue with Billy that there really were no monsters in lakes or swimming pools, or that aliens from outer space which would kidnap you in the night really did not exist. Rather, as Billy's sense of self and security got stronger, these delusional fears would disappear on their own.

Forming relationships with borderline children is not an easy matter. Often they have received only negative reactions from grownups and subsequently are wary of contact with adults. Other children are so socially awkward and immature in their interpersonal relationships that they can only utilize others in a need-fulfilling way. The therapist thus has to be a source of gratification before he can exert any real influence. This is also true with healthier children, to an extent. However, with these more mature youngsters, gratification can take the form of praise for a board game well played, a drawing well executed or simply a good exchange of ideas with a sympathetic adult. With the more disturbed child, gratifications usually are geared to be more concrete and immediate. In Billy's case, he continued to express a desire to have something to eat, an inappropriate request in a 10-year-old child. The therapist took Billy to a local delicatessen and bought him a small sweet and a soda. This initiated a ritual, wherein Billy would get a soda and sweet at each session. Later, the outings were limited to Monday's session, where Billy would select his treats for the week as an effort to help Billy in planning ahead in a very concrete yet, for him, very important way. Other ways of forming relationships with such children through tangible props are to build models together, make drawings or scrapbooks together, or even to look over a child's homework. The point is that these children are not accustomed to just talking to an adult and cannot produce verbal material easily in a regular interview situation. Much more of an interchange can take place around a separate activity that is shared.

Perhaps this might be a good place to talk about the role of play with very disturbed children. I have not found it very helpful with children of school age or older. First, it is too often a solitary experience for the borderline child, rather than a mutual activity. Therefore, it isolates the child from the therapist rather than building a relationship. Second, play is so unstructured that it may awaken fantasies that are best left alone for awhile. Erikson (1950), in his concept of play disruption, has perpetuated Klein's observation that the play of a very disturbed child may be frightening and anxiety producing. By this Erikson means that play loosens up thoughts which are so threatening that the play has to be stopped abruptly. It is simply too scary. Third, in play the child remains in a world of fantasy, whereas with these children one wishes to emphasize the world of reality. Too often, this fantasy is their prime occupation at home at the expense of experiences in the real world. While such fantasy play may be useful for normal or neurotic children in compensating for the frustration of reality, for rehearsing adult roles or for expanding their cognitive horizons, in the severely disturbed child, fantasy play is too often a dead end. It is repetitive and leads nowhere because this very monotony is reassuring in a reality that is so difficult to manage. Therefore, while most of us use play to expand our awareness through the use of imagination, these children use play for security and thus limit their experience.

The third and last objective of the initial stage of therapy is to form an alliance with the family. Anna Freud has written of the important role of the parent in child therapy as follows: ". . . it is not the patient's ego but the parent's reason and insight on which beginning, continuance and completion of treatment must rely. It is the task of the parents to help the child's ego to overcome resistances and periods of negative transference without truanting from analysis" (1965, p. 48).

With severely disturbed children, the parents must do much more than insure the presence of the child for sessions. They have to be involved as part of a therapeutic team that will continue corrective support outside of the office. They will need to know a great deal about this child who has often been a puzzle to them and they will have to painfully examine their own feelings for a child who can so disrupt their daily lives. Of greatest importance, they will have to begin to understand the relationship of their child's withdrawal or outbursts to subtle changes of the level of tension in the household and how to correct and eliminate this escalation of tension. Finally, while aware of the limitations of the patients, the parents should seek out areas of strength or talent to encourage and reward.

The second stage of therapy may be loosely defined as "ego strengthening." This vague term means that inner controls and arrested capabilities are encouraged to develop to age appropriate standards. To achieve this end, one relies on the three S's—supervision, structure and support. It has been my experience that this can best occur within the context of a close relationship with the therapist. Only when a sense of trust has been established will the child accept an alternative view of his distortions and misinterpretations. This sense of trust and mutuality constantly depends on the therapist's ability to correctly assess the level at which the child is functioning from one session to the next. Ekstein has also beautifully described this technical difficulty in maintaining a therapeutic relationship. Let me quote one of his most instructive observations: "The technical problem for the therapist is to accept, understand, and respond to the child on whatever level will permit him to reach the patient without pushing him into modes of relationships for which he is not prepared" (1956, p. 363). One has to constantly estimate at what level the patient is operating on a certain day or hour and engage him at that level, but with the goal of bringing the patient to a more mature appreciation of himself and of external reality. Therefore, while acknowledging the immaturity of levels of contact, the therapist always tries to get the child to act in a more reality-oriented, age-appropriate manner.

As part of this overall process, the so-called conflict free spheres of the ego are expanded and developed. This aspect of therapy is extremely important, for it gives the child rewarding areas of activity upon which to build a sense of accomplishment and a more secure sense of self. These children often express odd or idiosyncratic interests; however any hobby or activity that is free from anxiety must be encouraged and shared. Billy became interested in collecting leaves and in photography. This gave him a rudimentary sense of order and of mastery over a segment of his life. Gradually, he enlarged these hobbies to include an interest in botany and movie-making, respectively. In later years, he used his interest in movies as a common interest with other children that allowed him to begin socializing without excessive fear. In turn, this enlargement of mastery eventually gave Billy the confidence to find a summer job in his early teens at which he performed adequately, greatly enhancing his self-esteem.

Another aspect of ego strengthening is the correcting of distortions. Here, as in most of the therapy, interpretations do not help and sometimes are incorporated into the pathological fantasy world of the child. We all know that the distortions originally arose out of fear and an inability to control the emotional correlates of experiences. The task is to make the child begin to see the world, especially the social world, as unencumbered by his misinterpretations. Therefore, rather than psychodynamic interpretations, everyday experiences are reviewed over and over again, with the therapist suggesting alternate interpretations. Taking Billy as an example, he could accurately perceive the behavior of others but mistook their motives. He interpreted his father's attempts at physical affection as aggression and would become anxious when his father hugged him. Partly, this misinterpretation was due to his father's being frequently angry and violent, so that Billy generalized his affect to all of his father's behavior, but also partly to Billy's terror of physical contact. While Billy and I dealt with his discomfort about closeness, his father agreed to show his affection in a more restrained manner, to which Billy responded. This vignette is illustrative, for the father did not realize that he was being too aggressive for Billy and felt rejected when Billy turned away from him. Similar misinterpreted experiences are dissected and examined over and over, with the child trusting the therapist's insights. As the child acquires a more secure and realistic grasp of his environment, he is encouraged to pursue more activities, which in turn are shared and evaluated with the therapist. This corrective process is analogous with what has been called "working through" with adult patients.

I would like to be able to present a section on the final stage of therapy, but in reality I have found that there is no final stage. With increasing mastery, security and control, the child will overcome his developmental arrests and begin to make real progress in catching up to his appropriate level of function. However, with each advance that the child makes internally, the environment will demand more as the child grows older. Each developmental task will bring new threats and new challenges which will often require therapeutic intervention. The onset of puberty in such patients may be an especially troublesome time as social development may not have progressed sufficiently to deal adequately with sexual feelings and physiological changes. At this same time, societal demands for closer relationships outside the home, for more responsibility in school, and for greater self-reliance and conformity also contribute to renewed feelings of inferiority, inner tension and alienation. Thus, in the long run, therapy should continue until adolescence, at which time the youngster will have consolidated a sufficient sense of self to confront reality without recourse to self-defeating symptomatology. During periods of low stress, the frequency of sessions can be decreased and therapy may consist of merely reviewing daily activity. However, the therapist should be ready to reinstate frequent sessions and to reinitiate the ego-enhancing procedures when the environment demands new behaviors that are beyond the child's emotional capabilities.

This is not to say that the eventual outcome is negative. If one can continue to treat a borderline child into young adult life, the youngster will often do very well. At age 18, Billy is no longer in therapy. He has graduated from high school and looks forward to a career in journalism. He has been able to master his parents' separation, his passage through puberty, and his being away from home for short periods. He has a few friends and is beginning to be interested in heterosexual relationships. He is totally free of the terrifying anxiety and paralyzing fears that for so long made intimacy intolerable, restricted his imagination and stifled his considerable intellectual endowment.

REFERENCES

1. EKSTEIN, R. and Freedman, S. W. "A Technical Problem in the Beginning Phase of Psychotherapy with a Borderline Psychotic Child," in: Gardner, G. E. (Ed.), *Case Studies in Childhood Emotional Disabilities*. New York: American Orthopsychiatric Association, 1956.
2. ERIKSON, E. *Childhood and Society*. New York: Norton, 1950.
3. FREUD, A. "The Assessment of Borderline Cases," (1956), in: *The Writings of Anna Freud, Vol. 5*. New York: International University Press, 1969.

4. FREUD, A. *Normality and Psychopathology in Childhood*. New York: International University Press, 1965.
5. GOLDFARB, W. *Childhood Schizophrenia*. Cambridge: Harvard University Press, 1961.
6. GOLDSTEIN, W. *The Organism* (1939). Boston: Beacon Press, 1963.
7. PINE, F. "On the Concept 'Borderline' in Children," *Psychoanalytic Study of the Child, Vol. 29*. New Haven: Yale University Press, 1974.

Chapter 3

The Psychotherapy of Severe Depression

Silvano Arieti, M.D.

In these late 1970's, when so much is said and written about depression as a catacholamine disorder, when the condition is generally treated with tricyclics and MAO inhibitors, when a prominent psychiatrist and a leader in the fight against depression states that a pill is the most effective method for changing the human being from sad to glad, my voice is one among the few to reaffirm the importance of psychological factors both in the etiology and the therapy of this common condition.

In over thirty years of clinical experience with depression, I have never seen a case about which I could say that there was no psychological factor involved. I have never seen a patient about whom I could say that his depression was unrelated to his prior anguish, or about whom I could say that his depression came from nowhere and its origin had to be sought exclusively in a metabolic disorder. And yet, I want to stress that my experience has been predominantly with cases of severe depression, called by many others, not by me, endogenous depression.

In the present paper, I shall deal only with these severe or psychotic depressions. My stress on the psychological factors does not implicitly exclude other concomitant causes. Nor does it imply a rejection of drug therapy. I myself prescribe drug therapy to some, although I consider it a treatment for symptoms and of only moderate effectiveness in severe cases. I believe that anything that can even partially relieve the terrible suffering of the severely depressed patient is to be welcomed and greatly appreciated.

Although I recognize that my theoretical inclination and my personal clinical experience have influenced me, I nevertheless think that I can make the following statements with a fair degree of objectivity: One, indications for psychotherapy exist in every case of severe depression. Two, the intensity of the depression should not deter the therapist from making psychotherapeutic attempts. Three, concomitant or prior drug therapy does not make the patient less accessible to psychotherapy, except in cases where antidepressants or a combination of antidepressants and neuroleptics are used in massive doses. Four, drug therapy may have much more rapid action than psychotherapy in ameliorating the distressing symptoms, but it does not modify the basic structures of the personality which rendered the patient highly vulnerable to depression. Five, prior use of electric shock treatment does not make the patient less accessible to psychotherapy. However, during the period of forgetfulness, mild confusion, and other organic effects which follow ECT treatment, psychotherapy cannot and should not go beyond a superficial, supportive role. Six, psychotherapy becomes a necessity when drug therapy and ECT therapy have been ineffective, when the syndrome keeps recurring in spite of these treatments, or when the patient refuses to try physical therapies again. Seven, psychotherapy should be instituted in patients whose acute attacks have ended spontaneously. In these cases the aim is to make the reoccurence of the attacks less likely.

Before I can describe some aspects of a psychotherapeutic approach to the severely depressed, I must outline some psychodynamic views of depression on which this approach is based. Time limitations compel me to select only the salient parts of a long procedure which has been described in a recently released book by Jules Bemporad and myself.

The patient who becomes severely depressed cannot put into operation the mechanism adopted by a normal person who recuperates from a feeling of sadness, grief, bereavement. For example, a normal individual hears of the unexpected death of a person he loves. After he has understood and almost instantaneously evaluated what this means to him, he experiences shock and then sadness. For a few days all thoughts connected with the deceased person will bring about a painful, almost unbearable feeling. Any group of thoughts even remotely connected with the dead person will elicit sadness. The individual cannot adjust to the idea that the loved person does not live anymore. And since that person was so important to him, many of his thoughts or actions are directly or indirectly connected with the dead person and therefore will elicit sad reactions.

Nevertheless, after a period of time that individual adjusts to the idea that the person is dead. By being unpleasant, sadness seems to have a function—its own elimination. It will be removed only if the individual is forced to reorganize his thinking to search for new ideas so that he can rearrange his life. He must rearrange especially those ideas that are connected with the departed, so that the departed will no longer be considered indispensible—that is, indispensible to the equilibrium of the psychological structure of the survivor.

Like pain, sadness thus stimulates a change in order to be removed, but it is a psychological change, an ideational change, a rearrangement of thoughts and clusters of thoughts. Eventually the actions the individual took will alter as a consequence of this cognitive rearrangement. In other words, with a normal sadness, after a period of slowness or inactivity that prevents quick responses, there is a reorganization of function, first cognitive and then motor, which aims at bringing about a return to a state of normality.

The person who becomes seriously depressed cannot use these recuperative mechanisms, cannot do what I call "sorrow-work." He finds himself in a psychological trap from which he cannot escape. The overpowering feeling of depression keeps in a state of unconsciousness, or deep unconsciousness, cognitive structures and patterns of life which started at an early stage. In other words, depression has among others, the function of repressing cognitive structures.

According to my studies of patients treated with psychotherapy, there is always a preceding ideology, or a way of seeing oneself in life in general, or in relation with another person, or with a goal to be achieved, that prepares the ground for the depression. Although it is true that the depressive affect prompts the person to search for and find pessimistic ideas that justify the affect, initially the opposite occurs. The patient's ideology preexisted, and was kept alive for a long time in conscious or unconscious form. Although the patient may have been aware of the importance of the systems of cognitive constructs, he was unconscious of their origin, of how much they involved, or of the ramifications, assumptions, and presuppositions in feelings connected with them.

These cognitive demands in most cases originate in childhood but continue to accrue throughout life. In many cases, these cognitive structures and patterns make the patient live not for himself but for another person, whom I have called the *dominant other*. The dominant other is represented most often by the spouse, less frequently by the mother, a lover, an adult child, a sister, the father. The dominant other may be represented through anthropomorphization by the firm where the patient works or by a social institution, a class of people, etc.

Some other patients live for an inaccessible aim which I have called the *dominant goal*. When the patient realizes the failure of his pattern of living, he also recognizes that he is unable to change it. Thus he finds himself in a state of helplessness and hopelessness. A frequent example is that of a woman who used to consider her husband a dispenser of love and affection, a protector, a friend, a partner in every respect. Now she has started to see him as an authoritarian person who imposed his rule at times in a subtle, hardly visible way, and at other times in a manifest manner.

The patient's own life, at first believed devoted to love and affection, is seen now as not genuine. The patient has been excessively compliant, submissive and accommodating. Depression following realization of failure to reach the dominant goal is more common among men. The patient realizes that he is not going to be a great doctor, lawyer, politician, writer, actor, industrialist, lover, musician, etc. But he cannot change the direction of his goal. If the goal is not achieved, life is worthless.

The limitations of the patient, determined by his rigidity and adherence to an inflexible pattern of life, do not provide him with alternatives. As in the patient who experienced failure in the relationship with the dominant other, the patient may visualize alternatives, but they either seem insurmountable or worthless.

In the cases to which I refer in this paper, sadness cannot be removed and is transformed into deep depression. When unpleasant ideas occur they are submerged by the wave of depression. The cognitive basis of the condition is repressed, but the painful feeling is very intensely experienced at the level of consciousness. This last remark may seem at variance with what we observe in many patients who express depressive ideas about the way they view themselves, the world and the future. Beck has carefully described these cognitive elements which keep the patient in a state of depression.

In my experience with cases of severe depression, these depressive thoughts are used by the patient to justify his preexisting depression. They replace much more basic and more intense depressive trends, which have to be studied longitudinally since they go back to the early life of the individual.

Now, the initial stage of treatment is the most difficult, and the most crucial. As a matter of fact, we can say that generally, unless an immediate and intense rapport is established at the beginning of treatment, the likelihood of having a successful therapy is considerably reduced. At the beginning of treatment, verbal contacts are hard to make, not because the patient is withdrawn, as many schizophrenics are, but because he is absorbed in his seemingly everlasting mood. The effort the patient has to make in order to communicate appears enormous to him and, what is more important, futile. He seems possessed and overwhelmed by feelings of futility, helplessness and desperation.

The therapist assumes an active role from the beginning. He is a firm person, who makes clear and sure statements and who asks very few questions, or none. He is compassionate, but not in a way that can be interpreted by the patient as an acknowledgement of his helplessness. Unless the patient voluntarily explains why he is depressed, no effort should be made to compel him to justify his depression. If he is severely depressed he will not be able to answer, and the renewed awareness of this inability will make him even more discouraged and depressed. On the contrary, the therapist may initiate conversation by saying, "Most probably you do not know why you are depressed. In my work, however, I have found without exception that there are reasons for every depression. The depression does not come out of the blue. The anguish and the suffering stem from sources that a person like you, at a certain period in life, cannot find out by himself. He needs help." When the therapist succeeds in establishing a rapport and proves his genuine desire to reach, to nourish and to offer hope, he will often be accepted by the patient, but only as a *dominant third*—a third entity or person in addition to the patient and the dominant goal or dominant other. Immediate relief may be obtained because the patient sees in the therapist a new and reliable love-object. Although this immediate relief may be so pronounced as to be mistaken for a real cure, it is only a temporary experience. It may be followed by another attack of depression if and when the patient realizes the nature and limitation of this relation.

The procedure of leaning on a dominant third may arouse objections on theoretical grounds too. In fact, we have seen how often the difficulty of the depressed patient stems from his dependence on a dominant other, and now we would encourage him to substitute for the dominant other a dominant third. In other words, we would not promote in him the assumption of an independent role.

This interpretation is correct. However, we must be aware that similar to what we do in the treatment of schizophrenia, at the beginning of therapy with the severely depressed the therapist cannot disregard the demands of the illness and act as if it does not exist. The first meaningful rapport with the patient must be made through the mechanisms that the illness puts at our disposal.

After the first stage of treatment, however, the therapeutic approach must be characterized by a relationship in which the therapist is no longer a dominant third, but a *significant third*; a third person who, with his firm, sincere and unambiguous type of personality, wants to help the patient without making threatening demands or requesting a continuation of the patient's usual patterns of living.

When the therapist has established a good rapport, he must aim at the quick discovery and understanding of the patient's basic drama. What is the loss that the patient has experienced and which has threatened him so much? Has the loss disrupted a life pattern so that the patient is no longer able to sustain himself, and habits, attitudes, ideas and feelings on which he has always relied? The loss may not consist of actual things or be connected with definite events but may pertain to the symbolic values attributed to these things and events. Or the event may seem insignificant to others, and yet the patient may have attached to it the meaning of loss of a hope, of a fantasy, nourished consciously or unconsciously, that has filled a great part of his psychological life.

Many therapists who are convinced that the so-called endogenous depressions are the result only of biochemical disorders are not attuned to detecting the occurrences of previous stressful events. Or, if they are, they look only for facts and not for symbols. On the other hand, we must realize that even when a stressful event has taken place, the event becomes important only in the context of the patient's history and special psychological picture. This point must be emphasized because just as there is a large number of therapists and patients who deny the importance or the occurrence of precipitating events, there is also a conspicuous number of therapists and patients who give exclusive importance to them. They focus on the events and do not adequately investigate the course of life as it unfolded prior to the occurrence of this specific event.

The death of a person very important to the patient, generally the death of the dominant other, may seem sufficient in itself to cause a depression. However, in these cases too we must explain to the patient in terms that he will easily understand, and at a time when he seems receptive to explanation, that the sorrow, although justified, is different from depression and not the only cause of it. Whereas sorrow and sadness are appropriate, consonant with the facts, uneven adoptive depression is inappropriate and maladaptive. The therapist must be aware that the crucial problem lies in the inability of the patient to sustain the sorrow-work after the event. To understand this crucial inability, a longitudinal study of the life of the patient is required.

Now, let us discuss therapy of the patient with a pattern of submission to the dominant other. In cases of patients with the pattern of submission and self-blame, one of the first therapeutic challenges consists of ascertaining who is the person with whom the patient is mostly involved. Soon the existence of the dominant other will be revealed. Often the patient will try to protect the dominant other and will say that there is nothing wrong with this person. Whatever is wrong is to be blamed on the patient himself. But once the therapist has been able to gather enough information, the relation of the dominant other must be interpreted to the patient. Step by step we must clarify to him that he does not know how to live for himself. He never listens to himself; he is never inclined to assert himself, but cares only about obtaining the approval, affection, love, admiration or care of the dominant other. He is incapable of what Bemporad has called "autonomous gratification."

For the sake of the dominant other, the patient has conformed to the wishes of others and has denied his own. He has even led himself to believe that the wishes of the other *were* his own. At times the fault of the other has been transformed by the patient into his own fault or flaw. For instance, the extreme thriftiness of the dominant other has been transformed into the patient's alleged largesse. The carelessness of the other has become the patient's fastidiousness or his obsessive behavior. In cases of married couples the dominant other's lack of sexual desire has become an exaggerated sexual appetite in the patient, or vice versa. The immoderate demands of the dominant other have been interpreted in terms of the so-called frigidity or quasi-frigidity of the patient.

The patient must be guided by the therapist to become aware of his personal wishes, and of the meaning he wants to give to his own life. This is not easy to do because the patient has denied and repressed his wishes. In many cases we have to reevoke the daydreams, aspirations and fantasies of childhood and adolescence in order to figure out what the patient expected from his life and what his life plan was.

As we have already mentioned, the dominant other is not necessarily a person, but may be the whole family, or a special group, organization or firm. The patient's relation to them must be reevaluated and possibly changed. After the therapist has made some headway in the patient's psyche, several developments may occur. The patient may become less depressed but angry either at the dominant other or at the therapist, whom he would like to transfer into a dominant third. The anger and hostility toward the dominant other, most frequently the spouse, is at times out of proportion. Once repressed or unconscious ideations come to the surface, the dominant other may be seen as a tyrant, a domineering person who has subjugated the patient. At this point, the therapist has a difficult task in clarifying the issues involved. At times the dominant other really has been overdemanding and even domineering, taking advantage of the placating, compliant qualities of the patient. Often, however, it is the patient himself, who by being unable to assert himself and by complying excessively, has allowed certain patterns of life to develop and persist.

I have so far referred to the patient as "he" or "him." However, I must point out that approximately two thirds of patients belonging to this category are women, and if the English language required that I refer to the most common sex involved, I would use the pronouns "she" and "her." Undoubtedly the improved attitude of society towards women's rights and needs will change the cultural climate or at least the frequency of certain developments. At the present time, the still-prevailing patriarchal character of society makes it easier for a woman to assume the attitude of dependency on a male dominant other, or even on a female dominant other.

By tradition, many more women than men have overtly or subtly been trained to depend on others for support, approval, appreciation. Some of them actually live a vicarious life. The fact that society and culture have facilitated these developments does not exonerate the female patient from recognizing the role she has played. By omission or commission, the patient has allowed the dominant other to assume that specific position in her life. Many husbands, certainly helped by the prevailing patriarchal character of society, are not even aware of having played the role of dominant other. When they come to such a realization they may try to deny certain facts, defend themselves as if they are being accused, and require psychotherapy or family therapy together with the patient. The same remarks can be made, although less frequently, for dominant others who are not husbands.

When the patient is no longer concerned with the dominant other in his recent role, treatment will make more rapid progress. The patient realizes more and more that he has not lived for himself, or even for the world, but for a limited audience—often limited to one person, the dominant other. There will be a gradual abandonment of this stereotyped way of living, less regret for what was lost and also a progressive enlargement and embracement of life's possibilities.

However, even at this point the patient may become easily depressed, since depression has become his fundamental mode of living. Depressive thoughts should not be allowed to expand into a general mood of depression, but must retain their discrete quality and content, which have to be analyzed. The patient must learn that because of this pattern of depression even innocent thoughts at times have the power to elicit depression. Little disappointments or losses which lead the patient to self-accusation, guilt or severe depression are actually symbolic of an earlier, greater disappointment or of a life-long disappointment. But now the early losses or the recurring losses are no longer likely to be repeated, because the patient is learning to assert and fulfill himself.

The handling of irrational guilt feelings is important in the treatment of many cases of depression, not only at the beginning of therapy, but even at advanced stages. Strong feelings of guilt tend to recur. The pattern that the patient has learned and repeated for many years of life is the following: guilt feelings *leading to* atonement *leading to* attempted redemption. By atoning, that is, by placating, obeying, working hard, doing his duty, denying himself, by wanting peace at any cost, he felt he could obtain the love, approval or admiration that he desired. But if he did not get it, he felt guilty again, for not having done enough, for not having atoned enough. If some energy is left it must be used for self-punishment.

The patient continues to feel, not in a clear but in a rather vague way, that enough punishment will make him acceptable to others and will restore a self-image acceptable to himself. The cycle thus repeats itself. The guilt feeling is often experienced for hating consciously or unconsciously the dominant other, in a way reminiscent of the sadistic trends that Freud described as directed by the depressed patient against the incorporated love object. Thus the greatest relief from guilt occurs when the patient has drastically changed his relationship with the dominant other. However, this pattern of guilt is so ingrained in many patients who present the self-blaming type of depression that other psychological mechanisms are often transformed to fit into this guilt complex.

The therapist will eventually learn to handle little relapses or to understand and explain psychological vicious circles which are formed, or stumbling blocks which are encountered and tend to reestablish a mood of depression. For instance, the patient may become depressed over the very fact that he so easily becomes depressed, and any little disappointment will trigger off this state of sadness or guilt. Again, he has to be reminded that the little disappointment is symbolic of a bigger one. Another difficulty consists of the fact that some clusters of thoughts seem harmless to the therapist and are allowed to recur. Actually they lead to depression because of the particular connections that they have only in the patient's frame of reference.

Eventually, however, the emotional pitch of the therapist will become more and more attuned to that of the patient. We must also remember that the patient who is familiar only with the *mood* of depression searches for reasons for being depressed and succeeds in finding seemingly plausible ones. The therapist involved in deep psychodynamic therapy should not be easily sidetracked by them. They are part of the manifest symptomatology, and their significance and use must be explained to the patient. We must realize, however, that these ideas may accrue a superficial layer of depression over the deep-rooted disposition to become depressed.

Now, regarding treatment of depression following failure to reach the dominant goal. When the therapist has ascertained that the depression followed the realization on the part of the patient that he has failed to reach the dominant goal, or that he is going to fail hopelessly in life, the psychodynamic inquiry which follows the initial stage of treatment is focused on why such a realization had such a strong impact. The psychological integrity of the patient depended entirely upon the fulfillment of a life plan, but it was only a narcissistic integrity. Deprived of this, the patient feels mortally wounded and deeply depressed.

Therapist and patient must come to a full understanding of how important the fantasized achievement was. How many were its conscious or unconscious ramifications? How big a place did the patient allow this fantasy to occupy in his psyche? Is it true that life without that particular fantasy has no meaning? The patient must be helped to find alternative paths. Is it really necessary to be a singer, a dancer, a successful politician, a big businessman, in order to find a meaning in one's life? The patient will answer yes, at least for him. In many other instances he will say that intellectually he knows that he should say no, but with the depth of his emotions he feels that the achievement of that particular goal is necessary in his case.

From his point of view he is correct. His self-esteem and self-identity depended upon it. He now feels cheated of his dream. We must help him realize that he started with a great demand upon life. Whatever the origin, this demand has become a false pride from which he has to be relieved. But his life is certainly more valuable than an ill-founded illusion, a fantasy which had reached a stage of pathetic naiveté. The disillusionment must be seen as an awakening, as a recognition of unfounded values and as the start of a search for new and stable values.

In many cases we succeed in ascertaining a specific and very important reason, an account of which the patient gave supremacy to the achievement of a particular goal, and this reason must be explained to him. In middle childhood, the future patient came to envision the achievement of a particular goal as a way of recapturing the love, affection or approval of the mother, or of whoever was in the role of the significant other. Later in life, the patient came to see the attainment of that goal as the only occurrence which would make him worthy of love and approval and would make him feel worthwhile. His life was previously experienced by him not as beautiful, but as a long tunnel with only one exit, one commitment.

The treatment of patients of this type entails a call for a different integration of values and habits and for a considerable change in character. Thus, it may be difficult. Just as patients belonging to the previously described group had to enlarge their involvement with people and change their attitude toward the former dominant other, this category of patients must acquire a latitude of choice towards life claims. Many of the modalities recommended for patients with a pattern of submission apply also to patients who are pursuing a dominant goal.

Time limitations do not permit me to discuss another important type of depression, which I have called the "claiming type," and have described elsewhere. I shall instead conclude this presentation with a few remarks about the advanced stage of treatment. At an advanced stage of treatment with any type of depression, therapy should consist of going over the patient's life patterns again and again and of explaining how his present dealings with life situations are often in accordance with the old psychogenetic mechanisms. Sooner or later, the patient who has by now understood the psychodynamics of his life history, learns to avoid the old ways because he recognizes them as pseudosolutions, futile defenses, and vicious circles.

In some patients the old mechanisms tend to recur even after they have been completely understood. As a matter of fact, even discussion of them may evoke strong emotions which are not in congress with the gained insight, but which are the usual affective components of the original symptoms. For even after the patient has understood the meaning of his symptoms and behavior, it is much easier for him to repeat the old patterns. It must, for example, be constantly pointed out to the patient that he should learn to ask himself what he wants, what he really wishes. Quite often his attempted answer will be only a pseudo-answer. He may say, "First of all, I wish peace. Then, I wish the happiness of my children." He must learn and relearn that peace at any cost implies satisfying others before oneself, and that even the happiness of one's children, although a natural wish of every parent, is not a wish predominantly related to the individual himself.

In other words, the patient must learn to listen to himself and to reduce the overpowering role of the other. At the same time, he must make a voluntary effort to develop inner resources. In the attempt to imitate others or even to surpass others in proficiency and technique, some patients do not rely on their own individuality. Instead, they work for the benefit of others or take flight into common actions.

They must learn that they too may have artistic talents. As a matter of fact, some very depressed persons have become able to transform their conflict into high forms of creativity. Creative upsurges in apparently uncreative, conventional depressive personalities are a good prognostic sign.

Other secondary recommendations may be useful in the treatment of the depressed. Except during the time when the depression is very severe, the patient must be encouraged to be active. Inactivity fosters the depressive trend. He must assign himself graded tasks. A daily program can be structured with the therapist until the patient is able to do so by himself. He must often be reminded that contrary to what he believed at the beginning of his illness, life changes; the depression lifts and gusto for life comes back. He must be told that the worst moment is generally in the morning when he wakes up, when the depressogenic thoughts tend to emerge fully to be soon repressed and replaced by a general depressive mood. Another characteristic which recurs quite frequently is the acquisition of a personality trait which is the opposite of the one the patient has relinquished. For instance, a formerly submissive patient is now assertive to a degree which is beyond the tolerance not only of family members but of what social customs require.

Orthodox psychoanalytic procedure with the use of the couch and free association is not indicated in the treatment of severe depression, even during the interval periods. Many failures in treatment of these patients are due to the adoption of classical psychoanalytic technique. Similarly, many therapists feel today that retarded patients generally should be treated with less frequent sessions, from one to three per week. Many patients, especially elderly ones, do well with one session per week.

In conclusion, the treatment of the severely depressed requires a substantial change in the psychological makeup of the patient. This change is indeed realizable but only with difficult and assiduous work. We do not ask the patient to give up his identity, but rather, whatever lie or impossible value has become connected with the unauthentic identity. We do not help a human being to lose a sense of commitment, but only the commitment that seduces and saps the self. Although difficult, the treatment may be successful and rewarding for patient and therapist both. It is hard to imagine something more gratifying than the fading of a seemingly endless sorrow and the dissolution of a pattern of living which had drastically narrowed a human existence. It is hard to imagine something more uplifting than the restored ability to look with hope at the array of life's infinite possibilities.

Chapter 4

Seriously Disturbed Adolescents

Derek Miller, M.D.

INTRODUCTION

The organization of this presentation is a little like the treatment of seriously disturbed adolescents: in dealing with a multiplicity of issues of varying importance one must decide where to put the weight of therapeutic intervention. This clinical paper will look at some etiological issues and suggest techniques for how intractably ill and seriously disturbed youngsters might be treated. There is a difference between disturbed adolescents, seriously disturbed adolescents and intractably disturbed adolescents.

Disturbed adolescence may be defined as occurring in those disturbed individuals who have successfully weathered the psychological storm of puberty (which should be considered separate from psychological development in adolescence), and who have become adolescent. They are sometimes able to use self-righting mechanisms. Many adolescents, perhaps ten percent of those who become disturbed, are able to either use a chance appearance of psychological support and psychologically integrate, or sometimes they receive relatively brief therapy and the developmental track continues. Of the fifteen percent of adolescents in the population who are disturbed, probably some ten percent do this.

Seriously disturbed adolescents do not do this as easily. For some youngsters the psychosocial processes that are required to support the adolescent process do not exist. For example, there are the youngsters who because of intolerable trauma when exposed to the abuse of drugs, continue to use these in a seriously regressive way for many years. Another group of young people for one reason or another does not get parental support. Support only by the nuclear family is not enough; adolescents who are not exposed to a social system which provides them with extraparental adults and peers cannot normally develop their personalities. These are often the children of mobile families and very often these children will present for help, apparently seriously disturbed.

There are significant developmental issues. Some human beings become pubertal but never become adolescent. They reach their teenage years, but they have had seriously disturbed childhoods. They either suffered from physical illness, a variety of neuroendocrine disorders or severe nurturing deficits which led to characterological distortion. These human beings react psychologically to puberty but it is quite clear that they had the same personalities prior to puberty, except for the physiological change and the psychological response to the physiological change; they take no significant steps toward autonomy. A severely obsessional eight-year-old is likely to be a severely obsessional fifteen-year-old. For better or worse, the child has coped with some of the psychological issues of puberty. He or she has learned something about body image, something about dealing with issues of physiological helplessness, but essentially all this has fallen in the service of the characterological difficulty which existed prior to puberty. The same goes for childhood schizophrenics. Children who become childhood schizophrenics, which typically appears just prior to puberty, deal with puberty but they do not become adolescent because they cannot tolerate the stress of implied separation. The same is true of some types of unipolar and bipolar illnesses. In childhood and adolescence, the latter are often not recognized. These children are often seen as characterologically disturbed prior to puberty and they suffer from the same characterological disturbances thereafter.

A special group of disturbed children who are not well treated become intractably ill. This morning for example, you heard of a case of a youngster who was "borderline" prior to puberty. It was pleasant to hear the optimism but there are a number of intractably disturbed children who are not successfully treated initially and who very often appear as more disturbed at fifteen than they were at five. The significant issue is whether or not the psychological difficulty was treated successfully before puberty.

One interesting aspect of adolescent disturbance is that it would appear that the severity of problem presentation does not necessarily relate directly to the severity of the underlying illness, although the severity of the problem and its effect on others, as well as on the adolescent, significantly influences outcome. Most adolescent disturbances present as behavior disturbances, and a number of issues are important in terms of understanding intractability. Sometimes the symptoms that youngsters develop give them a pathological, instinctual gratification, and personality development is arrested. For example, it may be so satisfying to smoke marijuana that it seems to the boy or girl that there is no reason then to do anything else. These children very often become intractably ill because they cannot give up the drug. Alternately, they may not be able to abandon the gratification of tormenting their seemingly powerful parents. Sometimes they cannot give up theft; or they cannot abandon the power associated with suicidal threats. The threat to kill oneself gives individuals an enormous sense of omnipotence. Thus, the way a problem presents may make for intractability. Problem presentation may not only affect the personality development of a child, it may also confirm the child's disturbed view of the world.

HELPLESSNESS AND PERSECUTION

A generic issue in dealing with the disturbed adolescent is helplessness. Most seriously psychologically ill adolescents—the depressed, schizophrenics, those with character problems of a variety of types, those suffering from chronic psychosomatic illness—are dealing with problems of autonomy. Those who cannot individuate have to deal with a pervasive sense of helplessness. Along with helplessness goes a perception that the world is tormenting and persecutory. In the normal pubertal adolescent, often when parents are being perfectly reasonable, the youngster may respond as if they are highly persecutory. Typically, in middle-class culture, the child rushes to his or her room, announcing that never has an individual been so misunderstood. The benign intent of the authority figure is misunderstood and the child experiences persecution. Disturbed adolescents who have some capacity to appraise reality tend to have the confused feeling that the world is not as persecutory as they feel it to be. They then manipulate the environment in order to make it persecutory. If they can succeed with this, they then get a perception that they know where they are. Through this projective identification others are made persecutory and a bizarre sense of mastery, precisely what the seriously disturbed adolescent feels is needed, is obtained. The result of the problem presented is that, on the one hand, adolescents can get instinctual gratification from their symptoms, and on the other, their symptoms can be used in the service of making the world persecutory. These help to create a situation in which symptoms become part of a phenomenological psychosocial homeostasis.

SOCIAL SYSTEM COMMUNICATION

Residential care, individual therapy and family work all communicate to clients, implicitly and explicitly. Disturbed adolescents pick up the implicit environmental messages and, since these tend to be consistent, conform to these. Adelaide Johnson, in discussing the psychotherapy of sexually confused individuals, makes the point that they will often act out the unconscious wishes of the parents. Aichorn demonstrates that delinquent adolescents may play out the unconscious wishes of therapists.

Almost every communication from a social system to a child carries two messages: the overt and the covert. Simplistically, it is all too common to shout, "Don't shout!" In effect, the child is being told that it is all right to shout but one must be bigger and better at it. The messages that environments, whether families or therapeutic systems, send to children consistently indicate expected behavior of which individuals are unaware. For example:

> The family of a boy bitterly complained that he was delinquent. The father, who found cocaine in the house, threw it away. The father also made it clear to his son that he, himself, was cheating on his income tax; yet the father was bitterly persecutory of his son because the boy broke the law.

In family work with disturbed adolescents, families need to understand their techniques of communication and ways in which they convey mixed messages about behavior; in environmental settings, the same is necessary with staff.

DISTURBANCE AND PERSONALITY DEVELOPMENT

The care of the causes of illness does not necessarily resolve the personality difficulties that have developed because of the child's previously excessive symptomatic response to the perception of stress. Many characterologically disturbed adolescents suffer from a variety of neuroendocrine disorders. The failure to adequately treat the neuroendocrine disorder makes successful psychotherapeutic intervention very difficult. However, merely to treat the neuroendocrine etiology of the disturbance does not necessarily resolve the persecutory disturbance. The child may have learned techniques of relating to the world which maintain psychological homeostasis that is potentially distorted because of brain biochemistry. This may lead to a characterological disturbance. To avoid intractable illness, the etiology of illness, both neuroendocrinological and psychological, must be differentiated. Schizophrenic adolescents are highly intolerant of separation. This is because when an adolescent becomes schizophrenic, separation arouses intense persecutory anxiety. Schizophrenia is also an illness of longer duration than would appear on the surface. Before the appearance of acute disintegration, there is a prepsychotic phase of the illness. The psychotic phase of the illness, which it apparently starts, is followed by a postpsychotic phase. When the effects of the postpsychotic phase are not recognized, particularly on cognitive development, the illness may become intractable. This is also likely when therapists are changed. Intractability in this illness is often an iatrogenic phenomenon. There are multiple reasons for this. One schizophrenic episode can create cognitive regression and in particular this applies to formal thinking. A bright, academic individual who is no longer capable of abstraction at the age of fifteen, sixteen or seventeen can no longer function as before at school. If this is not recognized, and adolescents do their best to hide it, in the postpsychotic phase of this illness the adolescent becomes persecuted by both teachers and parents who complain of poor performance. Thus, the adolescent is reexposed to stress. Many of these young people are quite properly on tranquilizers. Under stress, further disintegration is likely. Particularly if there has been a change of therapists, the dose of tranquilizers commonly is raised. The adolescent is forced into an increasingly regressive stance, so a chronic personality disorder on top of a chronic neuroendocrine illness is created. The youngster is then thought to be suffering from an intractable process schizophrenia which becomes a self-fulfilling prophecy.

Many professionals still do not recognize that a significant number of character-disordered children are suffering from depression. Sometimes there is a clear depressive equivalent which may present itself in adolescents as a monosymptomatic behavior disorder. Children who present with a monosymptomatic behavior disorder should be considered as suffering from a possible unipolar illness equivalent. Children who suffer from affective storms may be suffering from a bipolar illness equivalent. If these are recognized and the child is given an appropriate drug, the extraordinary complexity of the therapeutic process is demonstrated.

A particular problem of psychopharmacology in the adolescent age period is that adolescents project omnipotence onto therapists and look for magic answers, as do their parents. Psychopharmacological treatment implies, as an implicit message, that magical treatment is possible. On the other hand, psychotherapy says there is no magical answer. This differentiation needs to be clarified with the patient when psychopharmacology is used, particularly with outpatients. If it is not, then the youngster is likely to drop out of treatment.

Another problem in this age group relates to ambivalence about omnipotence; adolescents who cannot bear the experience of helplessness, which is often felt as being reinforced by external control from outside, commonly refuse to take medication. Adolescents in this age group who are assisted by medication, who previously did not reach psychosocial adolescence and who became adolescent in treatment, may relate to a therapist as if he or she were a parental equivalent. They then refuse medication as a way of establishing autonomy.

Insofar as the use of appropriate medication for most behaviorally disturbed adolescents is concerned, a particular problem is that most never see psychiatrists at all. The most disturbed adolescents in our society are generally treated in the correctional system by social workers, clinical psychologists or youth workers. Most of these professionals have no significant training in understanding neuroendocrinology, or even the psychological effects of puberty.

The processes of psychological splitting are present in normal adolescence and need to be understood along with the development of intractable illness. Prepubertal children also normatively make splits and use the healthy nuclear family for support against splitting. To simplify: A child comes home from school and states "I hate my teacher." A good parent does not reply "You do not hate the teacher; you love the teacher." If this is done, the child feels alienated from his own experience. A good family hears the child express hate, listens, absorbs the concomitant tension and, as it were, gives the child back a sense of support. Winnicott had the idea that in holding a baby, a good mother absorbs tension and anxiety from the infant and restores a feeling of nurturance. In latency, a child can bring hatred home to the nuclear family, have it absorbed and then the child is able to function in the world. In adolescence, this process ceases to be possible, because to bring home a split implies dependence and abandonment of the attempts at autonomy. What the boy or girl then does is use his or her relationship with other social systems, extraparental adults and peers to absorb splitting. However, the problem of peer absorption of splitting is that peers reinforce the split. Peers generally do not say, "Really, the math teacher is a nice guy." They have to say, "Yes, I agree with you. He is a son-of-a-bitch." The tendency is that the split is reinforced and this may be felt as so intolerable that varieties of regressive and aggressive behaviors occur in attempts to relieve intrapsychic tensions.

Parents often can no longer tolerate not being the recipients of the child's splitting because they feel devalued and useless. To deal with this the parents tend to become coercive or rejecting. A similar problem occurs in the treatment of seriously disturbed adolescents. The social systems, typically schools and hospitals, absorb adolescent splitting. Often, individuals within these systems cannot tolerate being hated and the split in adolescence means that while they are hating, they cannot also love.

AMBIVALENCE AND SOCIAL SYSTEMS

Hatred is psychologically exquisitely painful to both donor and recipient. The more disturbed adolescents are, the more unable they are to feel any ambivalence. They constantly project their hatred onto therapeutic staff, who may then respond by becoming highly coercive. The more seriously disturbed the adolescent is, the more likely therapeutic systems are to become coercive or punitive. For example: standard hospital treatment for seriously disturbed adolescents commonly includes techniques of isolation, strap and chemical restraints.

The ego functions of severely disturbed adolescents are highly fragmented. Isolation rooms are euphemistically described as "time out areas" in which the adolescent is supposed to think about his or her situation. Isolation either reinforces fantasy or produces a regression which does not enhance personality functions. If seriously disturbed adolescents are isolated from nurturing support within which control is possible, they then become developmentally more disturbed.

INTRACTABLE DISTURBANCE

In intractable disturbance in adolescence, the individual can no longer make the move to preadulthood. Adolescence is the end of preadulthood, and the successful mastery of adolescent tasks makes possible the move into early adulthood. Intractability may be caused by a failure in the ability to resolve the psychological issues caused by an incapacity to be ambivalent, and the consequent splitting, projection and resulting coercive staff responses. Secondly, there may be a failure to make adequate neuroendocrine diagnoses.

Serious psychological illness creates a situation in which the nonspecific developmental needs of the individual are not met, either because supplies are not offered by the social system in which the individual lives or because the ability to internalize appropriately is lacking. All human beings have nonspecific needs which must be met if personality development is not to be impaired. Marijuana dependence may mean that a boy or girl may spend four or more hours a day getting "stoned," two hours a day discussing the drug and two hours a day acquiring it. The average adolescent who is highly dependent on marijuana may spend eight hours a day of his or her time in acquiring and using the drug. The psychological situation underlying drug abuse is the experience of boredom and emptiness. The physiological experience is the presence of the breakdown products of alphahydrocannibinol in the central nervous system because the half-life of the drug is larger than the gap between intakes. The complaints of emptiness, nothing meaning anything, and boredom are the depressive equivalents in words. In addition, the individual's capacity to be creative is impaired.

Such seriously disturbed adolescents lose their capacity for creativity and thus the experience of boredom and emptiness is reinforced. An additional, common side effect of serious adolescent illness is the interruption of cognitive development. The capacity for formal thinking may be temporarily lost if it previously developed and the capacity for academic learning is interfered with. In therapeutic interventions with seriously disturbed adolescents, specific interventions that are required may be initiated, but if the nonspecific interventions that are required (for example, to reinforce creativity and assist cognitive growth) are not undertaken, specific treatment is less helpful. It is very rare in the families of seriously disturbed adolescents that there is any attempt to do more than insist that the children go to school or watch television. The same is often true of therapeutic systems. Creative ability may disappear in very sick children and it is not enough to assume it will automatically return with the resolution of the disturbance.

Intractability may be created by a therapeutic failure to meet nonspecific developmental needs. The most intractably ill children tend to end up in residential care. Most residential care systems are psychologically depriving insofar as these needs are concerned. Bettelheim defined "institutionalization" as the creation of an emotional deficiency disease. The most seriously disturbed adolescents who require residential care are most likely to be exposed to this experience. The use of television in such settings demonstrates the point in residential treatment. The television set has become a way in which interpersonal experiences between people are minimized. Television reinforces passivity and lack of communication between people. Without television, care staff have to be creative in planning with the children, because left to their own devices, disturbed adolescents become highly disruptive.

Other nonspecific needs that are not well met have to do with exercise and activities. In many residential institutions there is a failure to recognize that growing adolescents need to eat after five or six o'clock in the evening as a simple physiological issue. It is difficult to find funds to take children to plays, concerts, and so forth. Occupational therapists often seem disinterested in what happens to adolescents after four or five o'clock in the afternoon. The compartmentalization of disciplines into separate and uncoordinate turfs does not assist in meeting their needs.

PSYCHOTHERAPY

The planning of the time, frequency, and technique of psychotherapy leaves much to be desired. The prescription of "group therapy" means only that a group of people are present with one or more therapists; it says nothing about technique or frequency. Family therapy means only that a family is present with one or two therapists. Individual psychotherapy means one patient with one therapist. Different syndromes require different types of psychotherapy. The forty-five or fifty minute hour may be totally inappropriate for some adolescents because seriously ill young people often cannot pay attention for more than twenty minutes. In our setting, whatever the intent, the more disturbed the adolescent is, the shorter the time is that the individual spends in a session. This is not necessarily because of the therapist's problems. A good psychotherapist senses the amount of time a child can use and does not insist that the seriously disturbed child attempt to do more.

Schizophrenic adolescents, when they are most disturbed, may be seen daily for about fifteen or twenty minutes. As they reintegrate from the acute psychosis, they can then use periods which vary from thirty to forty-five minutes. The prescription of therapeutic frequency is also often inadequate. The reason for prescribing five, three or one session per week is vague. Prescribing once-a-week psychotherapy, simply because that is the only time available, shortchanges the individual.

Expressive therapy is generally not a rational prescription for a concrete thinking, seriously disturbed adolescent. To such a patient, an interpretation may mean "You do not think I am saying what I am saying; you think that I am saying something else." For concrete thinking adolescents, an interpretation may become a psychological persecution which alienates them from themselves. Interpretations should be made only by people who are qualified to make them. Parents and child care workers should not make interpretations. If a child does not experience anger, it is difficult for them to be told by child care workers that they are angry.

Further problems in adolescent treatment are produced by conflict between the law and psychiatry. In many states, adolescents are seen as needing hospitalization only if they are ready to kill themselves or somebody else. A classic evaluation of one insurance carrier is "the mere fact that this boy is likely to commit matricide does not, in our opinion, justify his hospitalization." Society seems to have an implied hatred of children. The constant alienation of its resources affects the way care is delivered and reinforces the production of intractably ill people. Physicians are not psychological islands; psychiatrists live under negative social system pressures, and apart from the internal pain of dealing with children who constantly make the therapist feel useless, social systems pressures become a major problem in dealing with intractably ill and seriously disturbed children.

Chapter 5

The Intractable Borderline Patient: Treatment Considerations

Gerald J. Sarwer-Foner, M.D.

INTRODUCTION

Too many use the term *borderline* in a very loose, generally descriptive, but not specifically diagnostic, sense to delineate a large spectrum of latently psychotic patients whose symptomatology does not at a particular point reach psychotic proportions, or whose psychotic episodes are of short duration (5, 12, 27) and end with nonpsychotic, often characterologic, defenses (2, 4, 5, 7, 8, 14, 21, 24, 43, 47, 48, 49, 51, 55).

In this presentation, the author is dealing not with these cases, but with patients suffering from a character neurosis or personality disorder called "borderline personality organization" by Kernberg (15-18) and also delineated by Grinker et al. (9).

The issue of what borderline personality organization is clinically and psychodynamically—which factors enter into this diagnosis, its treatment, and what difficulties tend to make some of these patients intractable in a treatment situation, rather than smooth flowing and tractable in treatment—will be discussed. One should point out that only some borderline patients in treatment are definitively intractable, while others, properly treated, respond with gratifying progress over time.

The disease is a character neurosis or character disorder in its essence, and this by definition implies (and the implication is borne out in the treatment reality) that it is difficult to change established characterological ego defenses, and that changing these takes skilled treatment applied over a long time. This fact having been stated, it is nevertheless true that some patients are treatable, while others with whom one attempts treatment become the intractable or analysis interminable type of patient.

The Setting and the Clinical Spectrum of Patients

If one has worked in all types of psychiatric settings, one's view of the clinical range represented by the borderline patient is broader than the range of clinical tableaus seen by those who only do office practice. (The author has discussed this elsewhere (44, 45).)

What Is Included in the Various Uses of "Borderline"?

The term "borderline" is used in two very different senses. It is used as a rubric or general phenomenological classification in the descriptive, but nondiagnostic, sense to indicate a very diverse group of patients whose symptoms and natural course indicate that they float between the psychoses and the neuroses. Used in this way, it is an overall, nondiagnostic generalization about patients with multiple categories of symptomatology, which in their intensity, severity and duration float between the psychotic and the neurotic. It is also used nondiagnostically by some as a synonym for the latently psychotic (4-7, 11-14, 20, 21, 31, 37, 57).

The second use of the term "borderline" is in a much more specific diagnostic sense. It can be seen in the pioneer categorization of Roy Grinker and his colleagues (9). Grinker's study described patients with "anger as the main or only affect, defect in affectional relationships, absence of indication of identity and depressive loneliness." He defined four subgroups:

1) the "psychotic border," characterized by inappropriate or negativistic behavior and affect towards other patients and hospital staff; 2) the "borderline syndrome," characterized by negativistic and chaotic feelings and behavior, contradictory behavior, and a strong potential for acting-out; 3) the "adaptive, affectless, defended 'as if' person," characterized by a superficial adaptability but an affective deficiency; and 4) the "border with neuroses" representing childlike clinging depression.

Borderline patients in Grinker's study did not present disturbances in intellectual or associative processes, aggressive thinking, delusions, hallucinations, or defects in connotative language that schizophrenic patients show. Grinker and associates also felt that the "depressive aspects" seen in the borderline as affect were not altogether similar to those seen in the neurotic depressive reactions.

The Borderline Personality Organization

The work of Otto Kernberg (15-18), based on material obtained from psychoanalytically-oriented or psychoanalytic interventions, enables a specific psychodynamic diagnosis to be made, that of a borderline personality organization. Masterson (33-36) and others (11, 12, 26, 44, 45) have confirmed this view. Kernberg has worked to establish relatively short interviewing scales and techniques which would permit, he feels, anyone familiar with these tools to evaluate a patient in a diagnostic interview and make the diagnosis, when it is appropriate, of borderline personality organization. Gunderson and Singer (12), using psychological testing techniques, have come up with six paradigms which they feel enable them to do the same thing. Kernberg feels there are good correlations between Gunderson's "Diagnostic Interview for Borderlines" and the work he has been doing. Later work by Kolb and Gunderson (24) on a semistructured diagnostic interview has also shown good agreement with some aspects of DSM-III criteria for borderline personality disorder (criteria 2-4) and with some schizotypical reactive disorder patients as well as some who have brief reactive psychosis (criteria 1). Here, however, they include many of the latently psychotic.

LATE MATURATION

We do not have statistically reliable data on whether the untreated or poorly treated borderline personality organization patient "matures" in his fortieth to sixtieth years. There is data that suggest that this happens in certain psychopathic and impulse-ridden patients, and there is data that this occurs with a large number of people suffering from criminality. Many of them later settle down and seem to have belated maturation. Some of these patients may in fact be borderline personality organization patients. There is some data, yet to be confirmed, from George Brooks's Waterbury State Hospital long-term hospitalized cohorts (3), now being studied more than 25 years after their discharge into the community under the protective aegis of that hospital, that a proportion of these schizophrenic patients do mature and over time seem relatively indistinguishable in social living from their neighbors who were never hospitalized for schizophrenia. There is, however, no clear-cut data that this happens in a reliable way with the borderline personality organization group of patients. I suspect that it must happen with some, indeed perhaps with many, but no one has, to my knowledge, studied them long enough to establish this as fact. Thus in the use of the term "intractable," with some of these patients we are really referring to different situations.

Inadequately Diagnosed and/or Inadequately Treated Patients

There are patients who are not treated or are inadequately treated. They are seen by the physician only when they present in a crisis situation—with a suicidal gesture, a decompensated depression, with agitation and aggression because they have lost their jobs, with some sort of acting-out behavior (drunk, disorderly, etc.), loss of a significant relationship (marriage, love affair, etc.), a bad social situation (loss of home); or they present with dissociated, anxious or depressive symptomatology, with or without acting-out behavior. These crises pose the problem of accurate diagnosis—i.e., is the diagnosis to be limited to the diagnosis of the crisis (such as, adult situational reaction, depressive reaction, transvestism in a passive-aggressive or passive-dependent personality, a suicidal attempt or gesture, a patient with a schizoid personality, etc.), or is one able to make the underlying diagnosis in those patients who show the core structure of Kernberg's borderline personality organization? The latter is the character neurosis diagnosis, with generalized, predictable implications for its treatment course in the transference, and overall predictable implications for the countertransference pressures that will occur if one takes these patients into longer-term, intensive, psychoanalytically-oriented therapy or into psychoanalysis. If taken into psychoanalysis or long-term psychoanalytically-oriented psychotherapy, the aim is to change the character defenses and thus help the progression of a person with a borderline personality organization character neurosis into someone with more adult individuation, a better body image and identity, and therefore greater adult maturity.

Unbroken Symbiosis and Interminable Passive-Dependency Features

The second type of patient subsumed under the category "intractable" in a treatment sense is different from the patients just described. These are patients one has taken into intensive psychotherapy or psychoanalysis with some neurotic or characterologic diagnosis (2, 4, 5, 8, 22, 39, 51-53) or patients for whom one has made an accurate diagnosis of borderline personality organization. In the treatment setting, however, as the transference evolves and the countertransference pressures develop, these patients indeed enter some aspects of intractability, either through the progressions and regressions of their ego defenses (their oscillations along their own ego defense scales) with production of marked psychopathological constructs (signs and symptoms), or, for other patients, their inability in the final phases of treatment to terminate treatment, and their clinging to the physician for what becomes, for the physician, an unendurably long period of time.

Sometimes, from the patient's point of view, the situation may seem to be helplessly enmeshing, with the patient not knowing what to do about the remnants of an unbroken symbiosis which has not been analyzed or which the patient cannot, as yet, give up. The patient presses onto the physician a "demand" (sent via unconscious or conscious modalities) for a life-long, unbroken (and never to be broken by the physician) relationship. Not surprisingly this can produce intense and worried responses from the physician, often leading to unanalyzable impasses. Many aspects of these situations are discussed in this paper.

GENERAL DESCRIPTION OF THE BORDERLINE PERSONALITY ORGANIZATION PATIENT AS A BACKGROUND TO DISCUSSING TREATMENT ASPECTS AND PROBLEMS

The Capacity of the Borderline Patient to Relate to Others

As Grinker (9) has pointed out, the borderline patients form a spectrum or range of conditions. Some common aspects of those patients who are most accessible to psychotherapeutic character-changing interventions will be described. There are some who are more isolated or so easily enraged and projective that they are not really accessible to major psychotherapeutic interventions. They are not offered it, or if it is offered they often refuse or cannot use the treatment. Nevertheless, it is important to understand those factors that are common to the basic core of Kernberg's borderline personality organization patients.

Those most commonly treated in the offices of psychoanalytically-oriented psychotherapists or psychoanalysts are usually phenomenologically in Grinker's "border with neuroses" category or are the "adaptive, affectless, defended 'as if' person"; occasionally they fit into Grinker's "borderline syndrome" category but much more rarely are they the "psychotic border." Thus most of those taken into office psychotherapy have considerable relational capacity, with certain peculiarities and difficulties.

Anal Fixations and Defenses

In terms of psychosexual development, the "average" borderline patient seen in office practice has achieved at least an anal level of integration (10, 42, 53). In many ways they have had a reasonable oral phase, where they received enough physical, and in most cases emotional, nurturing so that bonding to external reality and objects occurred (so that they would not be schizophrenic), and they knew that they would physically survive. They have at least some optimism about external object relationships, and have achieved the capacity to contact and enter into relationships with others, meld and fuse with particular people who send the right signals. Their intense need to find others to relate to, to meld with them, is all part of the fact that they have had a not unreasonable oral phase of development.

Many of these patients, indeed the majority who present for intense psychotherapeutic treatment, are fixated at an anal level of personality organization (10). Here the treatment issues involve obsessional defenses, ambivalence-ambitendency in thought and action, a variable persistence of magical thinking and feeling. These are present because the patient has integrated many aspects of the oral and anal stages into a partial sense of personal identity, but with much ego and identity diffusion for later phases of development, particularly the phallic and genital phases (i.e., they do not individuate as an adult person). This identity diffusion is a critical issue, is always present and is therapeutically troublesome. Here the issue of an integrated or less integrated physical body schema arises. The question is literally whether their physical boundaries are established and complete. Where do they begin and where do they end? Toilet training helps complete the child's sense of control over his body and completes the physical body schema in that sense. In learning control over his sphincters he completes his sense of bodily self-mastery and the feeling that the body is physically his.

On completing toilet training, a sense of *organic body schema*, or completeness, is achieved—i.e., where one begins and ends in an organic sense. The child has not yet achieved his *body image*, i.e., has not yet added a sense of personal, cultural (including race, family romance, nationality, religion) and sexual identity (this comes later).

The borderline personality organization patients are disappointed with their perception of their physical bodies, and therefore unremittingly grieving and mourning, without much hope of change in this—that is, depressed about their literal physical body structure and schema, for what they are is seen by them as not enough.

At the same time they struggle with the issue of control over the body, its urges, and its relationships (10). (The physician has to know how to technically analyze these aspects (10, 42, 44, 51-54, 56). These are important considerations in relationship to treatability or intractability.) Are they the master, the slave or the victim? Are they superior or inferior, above or below whoever it is they are relating to? This issue of control touches all relationships and tends to tinge the nature of their ego defenses, their hopes, their real or relative hopelessness about further progression and change.

Thus, the borderline personality organization patient has

progressed enough in his developmental capacities to form relations (44). Borderline patients can relate. They can seduce, they can engage, they can enter into complicated sadomasochistic relationships. They can engulf people in their complicated web of ego defenses. This is to say that they are able to put energy into interpersonal relations and into relating to the external environment. They are able to form human relationships and to focus their senses onto external reality. This gives them the capacity to test and taste external reality in many ways. They are thus capable of many aspects of clear, rapid and complicated cognitive functioning.

Since the Borderline Personality Organization Patient Can Relate, What Is the Problem with Such Relationships?

His relationships reflect the fact that by himself he is not an integrated, individuated adult whole, with an adult sense of personal identity. Rather, this type of patient unconsciously feels, and expresses symbolically, in many aspects of his significant human relationships, that he plus another equals a whole person. The "other," who when added to himself forms a whole person, is usually a symbolized significant other from past life or a real person in current life. This is usually a symbolized version, most commonly of mother, but sometimes of father, grandfather, brother, sister—some significant other of the past. Even when it is not in reality the mother, the person is cathected with the functions of a good mother. The borderline personality organization patient is therefore suffering from an unbroken, symbolically expressed and interminably needed symbiotic relationship.

Despite this only partially developed state of personal identity, he has progressed enough in his psychosexual development to ward off psychotic disintegration. Masterson (33-36) used aspects of Margaret Mahler's studies (28-30) of the processes of separation and individuation to describe some aspects of this pathology.

In terms of a patient's body schema, he cannot be satisfied with what he/she is. Before treatment, the reality does not matter. She may in fact be a most beautiful and intelligent girl, or he may be a handsome, able and intelligent man. In terms of his self-esteem, self-image and view of his body schema, he has to feel that he is incomplete in his self-image and self-esteem so that what he is, is "no good," and would have been better had he been something else. Since there are only two physical possibilities, male and female, such patients always demonstrate some confusion about or dissatisfaction with their bodily structure, as part of their sense of personal identity.

Understanding this helps the physician conceptualize the way this patient feels about penis envy, doubts about sexual identity, the adequacy of one's body, and confusion over heterosexuality and latent homosexuality. The poor, devalued self-image of the totality of one's body schema follows. Such a patient does not understand an accurate description of his own gifts, assets, real beauty, intelligence and attractiveness. He tends to devalue real assets, which are then relatively meaningless, because such a patient has a "secret" that the physician who is attempting to treat him does not know if he ignores these factors. The secret is that whatever he is, is not good enough, is not as it should have been. It makes him feel that he is not a proper adult with an adult sense of identity.

Such patients integrate the rest of their body image in much the same way, as a partially fragmented, incomplete image endowed with relatively low self-esteem and low overall value. They really cannot believe it is good, and they feel it is incomplete in its essence, leaving them without a full sense of personal identity. A poorly integrated intrapsychic representation of both organic schema and body image is thus formed and is part of their identity diffusion.

Protean Symptomatology

They thus can present with protean symptomatic manifestations which oscillate back and forth over a period of time, with relatively integrated or relatively shattered ego defenses. They relate to bits and pieces of themselves and others. It has already been said that these patients have achieved the capacity to relate to others. They can therefore initially relate in a seductive and, on the surface, often apparently healthy fashion. They can be characterized as able to attract an object relationship, but cannot hold it over time. They can attract and beguile; they can involve others in complex, oscillating, often sadomasochistic maneuvers. They can entwine people in dependency, in slave/master relationships, and they can be the slave or attempt to be the master, or a combination of these.

Their pathology results in their leading restricted lives and never achieving their full potential. Many of these patients aspire to be many things, but somehow fail in these achievements. Part of this is related to their incomplete body image. No matter what they are or who they are, they feel they should have been someone, or something, else in order to be complete. The reality of their talents and abilities is not, at the beginning of treatment, emotionally significant for them. In their minds, no matter what they are, the next challenge still brings forth the feeling that what they are is not good, or not good enough. The issue of achieving self-mastery is, for the majority of such patients, translated into anal struggles for control where their regressed ego defenses repeat the unbroken symbiotic fusion ad nauseum in their progressions and regressions. They cannot evolve from this symbiosis into integrated human adults standing on their own two feet. What they express in their lives and therefore in the intensive treatment situation is this struggle with themselves. This struggle is then projected onto you, the treating physician, and the patient fights you for who he is, what he is, and what he cannot get away from. One aspect of this, more central to many than to others, is that they are superior, inferior, etc. They go on at this anal level of playing with these character defenses, which shows their concern about owning, controlling, demanding, and making sure that no one else can interfere or change their manipulative defenses (10). This is where "they live"; this is "where it's at."

SPLITTING AS A CENTRAL CORE OF THE DEFENSIVE POSTURE IN DEALING WITH UNBROKEN SYMBIOSIS

Describing the above does not account for how it is they cannot individuate. What is it that stops the individuation? What is it that stops the progress? Kernberg (15-18) in particular, and later Masterson (33-36), Sarwer-Foner (44, 45), and others, have pointed out that the child who later becomes a borderline patient, and who is initially progressing reasonably well in his psychosexual development, is faced at a point in his or her progression with an attempt to progress more rapidly than the mother wishes or can then accept. It is as though the mother cannot accept that the young child who is fused, in a relative sense, with her and needs her to exist, is suddenly becoming more rapidly independent at a speed and rhythm for which the mother is not ready, and to which the mother has not yet consented. The child making this rapid progression towards greater independence is suddenly faced with the mother's unconscious, and sometimes conscious, resentment at the child's trying not to need her as much in this phase of establishing his or her secondary narcissism. Mother responds to this with rage, irritation, frustration and fury, and sends what to the child is a clear signal, "I do not approve of your attempts to progress and get away from me. Thus I will threaten or carry out withdrawal of my love; my feeling, caring, presence." It contains in a fundamental way the threat of final, absolute rejection and the ultimate threat of abandonment. This threat of rejection and abandonment is vital, since the child then feels his inability to successfully live without the mother—i.e., it threatens death, literal death and symbolic death, the death of the growth of the psyche and personality. This often occurs at the same time as the struggle of toilet training, in the second year of life, or as a regression to this phase in the oedipal period.

The child understands the threat only too well; if he displeases the mother (or in many cases some other significant family member fulfilling the mothering functions), she will abandon him. The child thus suffers from existentialist dread, producing intolerable anxiety that if the mother were to abandon him, he would die. This is true even if the child at the time has no clear concept of death. They do have a clear concept of being flushed down the toilet or of disappearing, of being thrown out, of being swallowed, projected, or being magically catapulted into the outer world/inner world, sweated out, coughed out, spit out, urinated out, defecated out destructively and abandoned. The child has by then had the experience that people can leave but come back. On some level, he understands the concept of what happens to the bowel movement when it leaves the body and goes away. Where does it go? Is it abandoned or does it go to join other good bowel movements? Within the psychic, symbolic representations of a child of this age, the possibility of abandonment is in magical ways well established and stirs up the existentialist threat of abandonment and death.

For most of the above-mentioned authors (15-18, 33-36, 44, 45), this is the central issue around which the child learns not to progress, not to individuate and separate. Instead, the child learns to stop progression at the first sign of disapproval by the mother or significant mother-symbol. In the face of the anxiety generated, the child, with its limited repertoire, does one of several things. It divides the existing undesirable quality and its affect in two: that which is needed and acceptable, and that which creates disapproval and threat of abandonment. This latter cannot exist, must not be inside one. This splitting of the qualities in a sensorial and emotional sense is literal; the affect that is linked with the quality is split along with it. The undesirable quality and its affect are projected out of the psyche and body. There they can be placed onto someone else, identified and recognized in that person. At the same time, the projected split element is unconsciously "living" in the person who consciously no longer has the quality of its affect and therefore feels he has not got the undesirable element, the "badness." This "bad" quality is then seen as coming back at the person who has just projected it out with the same force and intensity with which it was projected. He therefore feels persecuted, attacked from outside and pushed by the qualities which are not desirable in the person (47). This persists into adult life as a central ego defensive mechanism in borderline personality organization patients.

These elements of splitting, projection, projective identification, of feeling attacked or pushed (sometimes persecuted) from the outside, come home to roost in the transference reliving of these phenomenon in the therapeutic situation. This forms part of the core issue around progression and its difficulties. Thus, the handling of the transference reliving of these elements is a good part of what determines whether the patient progresses towards improvement, or develops some aspects of the intractable borderline patient.

In the treatment setting, the patient's transference unconsciously pushes the split, projected qualities onto the treating physician, in whom they are now identified. These mechanisms of projection and projective identification, with or without the other aspects of projective idealization or degradation described by Kernberg, are part of what pushes the physician's countertransference feelings into unconsciously determined responses. The patient emotionally interprets these as reliving exactly the patterns developed in the first relationships with the mother symbol that created these patterns. The way in which the reliving of the transference experiences and the countertransference pressures are dealt with by the physician and by the patient, individually and together, determine whether the treatment is successful or fails. Intractability can be one response to these factors.

Thus, using the splitting mechanisms, the patient is locked into an unconscious, unbroken symbiosis in which he and somebody else equals one. This produces the lack of personal identity, or of identity diffusion, described by all who have worked with these patients. These patients cannot work with an integrated sense of identity and self.

The patient uses splitting, projection, projective identification with projective idealization or projected degradation, along with the obsessional defenses of dissociation of thought and affect, denial, ambivalence and ambitendency, magical doing and undoing, as central core ego defenses enabling the patient to maintain the sense of ego diffusion and unbroken symbiosis, thus producing the character disorder called the borderline personality organization.

To sum up this part: Faced with the child's attempts to progress to more independence, the parent cannot stand the child's precocious attempts to leave it. The parent then sends a clear-cut signal of disapproval indicating withdrawal of parental love and affection, and indicating that the child will be abandoned. The child clearly perceives this threat and develops a build-up of intolerable anxiety. The splitting then takes place within this context, the undesirable quality and affect being projected, etc. The child very rapidly learns to fall back from this progression in the face of the mother's threatened withdrawal. The child learns, "I must not progress. I must never leave you, mother. I must never really be independent of you. I must never displease you. I must always oscillate back and forth to just where you want me to go, there and no further, because if I go further you will cut me off. I will be abandoned. I will have nothing. I will die." Thus, power struggles (10, 42, 43), manipulative control struggles, struggles to submit or dominate, to oscillate, and to subtly outwit are all part of the character defenses of the borderline and are relived in toto, ad nauseum, in the transference treatment situation. The transference reliving pushes the countertransference responses of the treating physician along the same lines. In this regard the magical aspect of omnipotent and anal defenses, of controlling, of turning into the opposite, of magical causality in which a wish is the same as an act has to be remembered. Such patients make little or no distinction between wishing to have you drop dead and you dropping dead. If you happen to drop dead it is "my fault" for wishing it. There is an enormous need to always identify new object relationships within any environment as exact carbon copies of the significant power relationships of their past. That is why the control and power relationships of the anal phase of the development experienced with their parents are important. Thus such patients beguile, seduce, and meet everyone in their environment with the same processes to be carried out interminably.

To sum up the main characteristics of the borderline personality organization character structure. Such patients have the capacity to have object relationships, in other words to use the senses to identify people and objects to relate to; and once they do so, they can invest energy into relating to them. They can beguile, entwine and see if they are superior or inferior. They use splitting, projection, projective identification (with or without idealization or degradation), and anal aspects of control to deal with these relations and their own affects. They have an inadequate body image. They are often in symbiotic fusion with another person, in which they plus the other person equal one, so that they cannot be totally individuated as a complete adult. They thus feel that they are not a complete person and that what they are is inadequate. They have fluctuating but relatively low self-esteem. They feel they are not particularly valuable, and they use denial, turning into the opposite, dissociation of thought from affect, ambivalence, ambitendency, and a causality using magical thinking, in which a thought or a wish is the same as a real external event. All of this oscillates back and forth between a series of ego defenses, with progressions and regressions around a mean point. This oscillation about an essentially nonpsychotic mean point protects them from severe psychosis but does not allow them to function as a completely integrated, individuated adult person.

Psychotic Patients in Remission, the Latently Psychotic, versus Borderline Personality Organization Patients

One must distinguish between: 1) patients who have been psychotic with schizophrenic illnesses, who have at least partially recovered and now have some level of partially disorganized ego defenses, but at a nonpsychotic level at the moment of examination; 2) other patients, latently psychotic as in 1) or not psychotic, who have weakened ego defenses and great vulnerability to developing a psychosis; and 3) the truly borderline personality organization patients, who are not psychotic, are unlikely to become permanently psychotic, but have ego defenses organized in this character neurosis. On the surface some of the symptomatology may look similar. The differences are, for teaching purposes, outlined in sections of this paper.

Some patients, with what the French author V. Magnan in 1886 (27) and many years later Henri Ey (6) called "une bouffé delirante" (acute delusional psychosis (13)) may form part of the spectrum of patients with borderline personality organization syndromes. (Other such patients are best seen as latently schizophrenic, schizo-affective or schizophrenic-paranoid type patients.) These are patients who develop a circumscribed, short-lived, acute schizo-affective type of psychosis, with vivid hallucinatory and delusional material. They present with great affect and good investment of affect onto external objects. These episodes are usually self-limiting (lasting a few days to two or three weeks) with generally a good recovery to their preexisting personality. The French authors have separated this as a separate diagnostic entity.

In North America we would characterize this psychosis as a short-term, limited schizo-affective psychosis belonging to the schizophrenia group of illnesses. The point is that some of these patients do develop schizophrenia (paranoid type) over time, while others, carefully examined, show features best classified as belonging to the borderline personality organization patient, once they are out of their acute schizo-affective phase of psychosis.

Some patients with psychosomatic conditions, described in the French psychoanalytic and psychosomatic literature in papers by Marty and de M'Uzan (32) as "la pensée operatoire" patient (literally, the operational thinking type of patient), deserve to be classified as borderline personality organization patients. These are the same type of patients classified as suffering from alexithymia in the North American literature by Nemiah and Sifneos (38, 50), and Krystal (25).

Thus, concretistic thinking, incapacity to consciously feel or express emotions, and an incapacity to use verbal symbols is seen. They send emotions down organically predetermined or biologically conditioned neuronal, hormonal, and/or immunologic autonomic nervous system pathways. When these patterns continue, they produce the tissue lesions of psychosomatic illness. A selected proportion of such patients belong to the borderline personality organization category.

The point that a primary diagnosis of an acute disease does not eliminate a secondary personality or characterological diagnosis should be remembered (e.g., acute depressive reaction in a patient with borderline personality organization or acute duodenal ulcer in a patient with a borderline personality organization).

Certain borderline personality organization patients regress when their defenses crumble with the development of a depressive illness. They then show typical depressive symptomatology including the state-bound level of consciousness, demonstrated in the "delusion of the eternity of the depressed state"(41)—the feeling that the depressive illness will last forever. Some of these responses are seen in decompensated reactions of borderline personality organization patients, while other depressed patients are without the borderline core. The presence or absence of the diagnostic features of the borderline personality organization distinguishes them. Some acting-out patients, adolescent or adult, with or without antisocial symptoms, can be classified here (51) if one finds the borderline core diagnostic points.

Treatability or Interactability in Psychotherapeutic Treatment of Borderline Personality Organization Patients

These patients demand the "presence" of the treating physician in the treatment. They want to see, hear, be able to look at—some would like to touch—the physician, although we do not permit this. They must have the physician "in their senses." It is only through the presence of the physician through these modalities that they are sure that the abandonment they fear has not taken place, or will not take place.

A pure, classic psychoanalytic technique is often relatively contraindicated with them. Classic analysis, where the patient lies on a couch unable to see the analyst often fails, because the analyst has not already identified the above-mentioned needs in these patients, the patient giving up the treatment with resentment and rage with the analyst feeling that no progress can be made after a variable time (six months to a year of work).

The issues involved in forming a therapeutic alliance have to be presented to the patient from the beginning. The physician has to verbalize the importance of the patient working to master what he could not up-to-then handle, and that the physician will commit himself/herself to work with this patient as long as is necessary to achieve this. Here, the patient in his turn is asked to commit himself to this process in associating to this material. In this initial approach of commitment to treatment lies the make or break of many of these therapeutic relationships. It is also the key around which the issue of intractability as an early issue emerges, since inherent in what I am saying is a promise that the physician is ready to work with the patient and see the patient through the therapy, which the patient can misinterpret in favor of treatment being an undetermined and interminable treatment course—i.e., "You will live with me forever, you will fuse with me, you will always be available to me; and if you ever try to leave me or let me go, I, the patient, will regress into my illness." The unconscious menace of this type of pressure on the physician is of course perceived by most physicians, at least unconsciously, and does not encourage most to work with this type of patient. (It is much the same problem that one faces with a schizophrenic patient in such circumstances—a much too demanding central core of testing and retesting, both in the therapeutic alliance and in the therapy (48).) Yet one has to say, that without this type of commitment on the part of the physician, and the resulting initial reality-testing and exploration of realistic arrangements with the patient for treatment, no adequate treatment can ever begin; and without this, treatment attempts are doomed to failure from the very onset.

Not all patients, who can be identified as borderline personality organization patients are prepared to make this type of commitment. Nor are they unconsciously confident that they can exact this price from the physician. This is particularly true in lower class psychiatric outpatient settings where the patients realistically feel that the treating institution does not, in most cases, offer much to begin with. Gerald Adler (1) is therefore correct (for many of these patients) when he talks about "the myth of the therapeutic alliance." He is incorrect, however, if by this he means that *no one* can form such a relationship with *any* borderline personality organization patient. For many patients with whom this area is carefully explored, it is possible to form a working alliance and a therapeutic alliance. This has been done successfully on many occasions, the therapeutic alliance being cemented and treatment begun. Adler is nevertheless correct for a category of these patients.

The physician must be "authentically" present in the therapeutic relationship. It is often best to have the patient sit up facing the physician, across the desk from the physician; or in psychoanalysis, if the understanding is that the patient will take the couch, to have the physician sit where the patient can see him for the first part of the treatment. In successful psychoanalytic treatment of a borderline patient, it is the author's preference as part of the terminating phase of treatment (which is usually long and difficult in its own right) to ask the patient, who by then understands both emotionally and intellectually what processes are involved, and has by then developed (through his thorough testing) a real trust in the integrity, character, persistence and good intentions of the physician, to now try to do analysis with the physician sitting behind the patient, so that the patient can no longer see him. This withdrawal of the visual image of the physician from the patient brings up again all the anxiety about disapproval, withdrawal, abandonment, but now with a stronger patient who has identified with the physician. This is worked through over an appropriate time and is a pertinent part of the terminating phase of treatment with these patients. The ability to deal with this successfully helps the patient go on to the next phase of further separation from dependency on the physician and to greater personal individuation of the patient, preparing for the inevitable termination of treatment.

The patient thus cannot stand in the initial therapeutic contacts an aloof, reserved, disinterestedly neutral psychiatrist—one who seems to the patient to signal "I do not care whether you do well or not; it is up to you. I am just trying to be helpful." It is very important that the physician present to the borderline personality organization patient, "I do care that you progress, but I put this issue on your shoulders, and hopefully you will progress with my help. I will be here actively working with you in the process of your progression."

It is important to understand that less intensive forms of psychotherapy, and the use of other therapies such as pharmacotherapy, partially succeed or flounder on exactly the same bases as described above. The difference in the therapies is that with less intensive forms of psychotherapy, or other therapeutic methods (19, 20, 40), the factors described here are often not identified completely, or at all, and are not analyzed or worked with in terms of the patient's character structure. Thus these constants apply to any form of treatment of an unsuccessfully treated borderline personality organization patient. Knowledge of the above and paying attention to it in detail will make more workable, and certainly less mysterious, an otherwise almost magically difficult "intractable" group of patients.

The ability to analyze these phenomenon and present them to the patient for the patient's consideration and work is crucial. As this is successfully done, what had been ego-syntonic, i.e., acceptable to the patient as his/her usual way of feeling, perceiving and dealing with these things, is turned by the physician's clarifying interpretations and confrontations made in the living, affective exchanges between them into areas worthy of affective study by the patient's observing ego. This results in the breaking down of dissociation, denial, intellectualizing, rationalizing, splitting and projective defenses. As this is done, areas of the patient's pathological character defenses, hitherto ego-syntonic, become ego-dystonic for the patient, who then, for the first time in therapy, consciously suffers pain from this pathology and becomes more emotionally, as well as intellectually, motivated for change. The patient's material, behavior and associations put automatic pressure, conscious and unconscious, on the physician to respond to the patient's tone and behavior. This automatically forces responses to the patient (unconscious countertransference responses) which push the physician in the direction of behaving exactly like the disapproving parent who in the first place inhibited the patient's progression toward adequate separation and individuation. The persistence and reliving in the repetition-compulsion of the patient's mostly unconscious, unbroken symbiotic relationship with the parental figure of his/her past is now relived in the present, with the parental figure of the physician producing the automatic, unconscious countertransference responses. This has to be meticulously psychoanalyzed, giving the patient the time needed to work through this material. Success in working in the here and now demands at this point in treatment the genetic reconstruction of the roots of these phenomenon. Here the physician brings the genetic roots and their reconstruction into the patient's present life, and into analysis of the current unmastered problems in the patient's real life. The author also encourages the patient to explore in free associations what his responses will be for the rest of his life, as he develops his real talents and abilities to individuate, grow and therefore be free to use and expand his real assets.

The successful handling of these phases leads to more tractable patients. Getting stuck, not being able to identify and therefore to analyze the true nature of the reliving of the transference patterns; or not being able to handle his own countertransference feelings, attitudes and behaviors lead to difficulties that vary from rupture of therapy with failure in the progression of the patient toward individuation to a more on the surface comfort for the patient and sometimes for the physician—an ongoing relationship, but here a therapeutic relationship that does not evolve toward further progression and cure. Instead, it produces a rather stable relationship and unbroken symbiosis, which is now gratifying to the patient, in which the patient takes care to be agreeable and pleasant to the physician on most occasions. Unless this is analyzed by the physician with the above-mentioned techniques, but working in the here and now as an initial step, further progression often does not occur, the patient here being indeed intractable.

TERMINATION PHASE

If one successfully survives the vicissitudes of the above-mentioned phases, the next great hurdle (and perhaps the greatest hurdle for many) in the treatment of the borderline personality organization type of patient is the termination phase of treatment. Here the patient can relive many difficulties, recapitulating the vicissitudes of abandonment and regressing from a primary partial progression.

Regression in the face of a threatened abandonment for having progressed is a major, initially egosyntonic character defense used in response to the patient's conscious awareness of a threat of abandonment (by definition the essence of the parental disapproval). The threat of abandonment is precisely what triggered the patterns of the patient's regression. Now, by definition, in the terminal phase of treatment one is living and working with the issue of termination and therefore, at one level, of abandonment. The vicissitudes of this process, if badly handled, lead to an intractable borderline patient and this is one of the commonest of crises seen. Here the intractability is caused by the inability of the patient to give up treatment, i.e., to break the symbiotic bond of the transference. As already stated, the comfort of this bond is in some cases also shared by the physician in the countertransference, since by then the patient and physician have shared many years of treatment. There has to have been something agreeable about the patient and the relationship, otherwise why would the physician have tolerated it for so many years even as a duty? The issues of the gratifying aspects of the relationship (and here I mean nothing professionally improper, but only the ordinary human meaning of therapeutic work shared for so long and the affective relationships that have developed in the process) have to be analyzed with great honesty and integrity. By then (after years of work) the patient is fully able to do this even though emotional vulnerability to abandonment and rejection remains a greater hazard for this category of patient than for many others.

The author will often introduce work in this area with a gradual removal of any parameters that may have been introduced when technically necessary. For example, if the physician has sat so that the patient could see him from the couch, this issue is now raised for the patient's consideration: Is the patient now ready to face up to the physician sitting (as in a normal analysis) behind the patient, out of the patient's sight? It is important not to impose this on a patient, but to present it as a problem to be solved together when the patient is ready.

In psychoanalysis, if the patient has never taken the couch but has always sat up, now that he/she is strengthened, the issue of taking the couch for a time may be raised. Unconsciously at least, the patient will understand that such issues are in fact harbingers, not of spring but of termination, even if the termination is still some distance off. Panic, anxiety, splitting, acting-out tendencies, accusations; some or all of the borderline defenses, with threatened or actual regression, will occur. The recurrence of some level of the original symptoms with which the patient entered treatment often happens here, and sometimes symptoms never seen before develop (46). This is the patient's way of saying, "I am as sick as the day you first saw me. How can you be so heartless as to think of leaving me?" These regressions are a specific reliving of the patterns of the regressive mode of the particular patient back to a symbolic relationship. Failure to properly analyze and work through these phenomenon makes the patient the interminable or intractable patient, while successful analysis, working through and progression lead to the next series of hurdles. The patient can only tackle them after he/she has identified with the benevolent strength of the physician, making it his or her own.

Once some of the above is successfully achieved, the physician raises (or the patient, himself, raises—often as a kind of testing trap for the physician) the question of how one will *eventually* end this therapeutic relationship? The author's technique with this type of patient is not to unilaterally set a date for ending therapy (as one can with a more normal neurotic patient), but rather to ask the patient to work along with the physician to decide as one works when the eventual termination date will be.

The author says, for example, "You have entered the termination phase which will take a certain time. Let us see how we can evolve toward it, you taking the time you need for doing it, as quickly as makes realistic sense, but with you and I, together, deciding when and how this is to be done." Full confrontational interpretation and clarification is done, usually linking the patient's emerging material in the present with all that the patient already knows and has experienced by having repeatedly worked through the various aspects and repetitions of these phenomenon in the long analytic work already done. Here, further progression is encouraged by a thorough analysis of the fantasies of progression as they occur in the patient. Successfully dealing with this leaves the patient to increasingly face, with lessening dread, the issue of individuating and standing on one's own feet. In the successfully treated case, there are by now many real, adult successes and developmental progressions confidently embedded in the patient's ego and character. The patient's identity as an adult is more solid, having through the years of work with the physician first introjected him and then slowly identified with the good, steady, mature, and capable aspects of the analyst, adding them to the good parts of the original partial identifications the patient already had with the good qualities of his own parents. Thus the patient is now much stronger and much more able to bring his real assets to bear on this problem.

As this is done, with full confrontational intepretation and clarification of what is still murky and unmastered for the patient, the patient is able, in a successful case, to terminate treatment. In those patients not able to handle this, and in those physicians whose technical skills fall short of helping some of these patients deal with this matter, this phase of termination is a quagmire in which the patient and the physician wallow, the patient becoming the interminable or the intractable patient. Badly conceived and carried out terminal attempts merely leave a sick patient with an unbroken symbiosis, angrily hurt, scheming, and acting-out to get back into therapy with someone, or in frightened and sometimes suicidal despair. In others, mishandling this leads not to rupture of treatment, but to a continuance of what then rapidly becomes a truly interminable relationship, which is terminated only by forcing the end of treatment or transferring the patient to someone else.

It is these many factors that make a patient intractable or tractable.

REFERENCES

1. ADLER, G. "The Myth of the Alliance with Borderline Patients," *Am. J. Psych.*, 136:642-645, 1979.
2. BRODY, S. *Passivity*. New York: Int. Univ. Press, 1964.
3. DAUM, C. M., BROOKS, G. Q. and ALBEE, F. W. "Twenty Year Follow-up of 253 Schizophrenic Patients Originally Selected for Chronic Disability: Pilot Study," *Psychiat. J. Univ. of Ottawa*, 2:129-132, 1977.
4. DEUTSCH, H. "Some Forms of Emotional Disturbance and Their Relationship to Schizophrenia," *Psychoanal. Quart.*, 11:301-321, 1942.
5. ERKSTEIN, R. and WALLERSTEIN, J. "Observations on the Psychology of Borderline and Psychotic Children," *The Psychoanalytic Study of the Child, Vol. 9*. New York: Int. Univ. Press, 1954.
6. EY, HENRI. "Psychoses délirantes aigues," *Manuel de Psychiatrie*, Paris: Masson, 244-254, 1960.
7. FEDERN, P. "Principles of Psychotherapy in Latent Schizophrenia," *Amer. J. Psychother.*, 1:129-144, 1947.
8. GELEERD, E. R. "Borderline States in Childhood and Adolescence," *The Psychoanalytic Study of the Child, Vol. 13*. New York: Int. Univ. Press, 1958.
9. GRINKER, R. R., Sr., WERBLE, B., and DRYE, R. C. *The Borderline Syndrome*. New York: Basic Books, 1968.
10. GRUNBERGER, B. "Etude sur la relation objectale anale," *Rev. Francaise Psychoanal.*, 24:138-160, 166-168, 1960.
11. GUNDERSON, J. G. and KOLB, J. E. "Discriminating Features of Borderline Patients," *Am. J. Psych.*, 135:792-796, 1978.
12. GUNDERSON, J. G. and SINGER, M. T. "Defining Borderline Patients," Am. J. Psych., 132:1-10, 1975.
13. HIRSCH, S. R. and SHEPHERD, M. *Themes and Variations in European Psychiatry*. Bristol: John Wright & Sons, 395-404, 1974.

14. HOCH, P. H. and POLATIN, P. "Pseudoneurotic Forms of Schizophrenia," *Psychiat. Quart.*, 23:248-276, 1949.
15. KERNBERG, O. F. "Borderline Personality Organization," *J. Amer. Psychoanal Assn.*, 15:641-685, 1967.
16. KERNBERG, O. F. "The Treatment of Patients with Borderline Personality Organization," *Internat. J. Psycho-Anal.*, 49:600-619, 1968.
17. KERNBERG, O. F. "A Psychoanalytic Classification of Character Pathology," *J. Amer. Psychoanal. Assn.*, 18:800-822, 1970.
18. KERNBERG, O. F. *Borderline Conditions and Pathological Narcissism.* New York: Jason Aronson, 1975.
19. KLEIN, D. F. "Psychopharmacology and the Borderline Patient," in: Mack, J. E. (Ed.), *Borderline States in Psychiatry*, New York: Grune & Stratton, 75-91, 1975.
20. KLEIN, D. F. and SHADER, R. I. "The Borderline State: Psychopharmacological Treatment Approaches to the Undiagnosed Case," in: Shader, R. I. (Ed.), *Manual of Psychiatric Therapeutics.* Boston: Little Brown, 281-293, 1975.
21. KNIGHT, R. P. "Borderline States," Bull. Menninger Clinic, 17:1-12, 1953a. "Management and Psychotherapy of the Borderline Schizophrenic Patient," Bull. Menninger Clinic, 17:139-150, 1953b.
22. KOHUT, H. *The Analysis of the Self.* New York: Int. Univ. Press, 1971.
23. KOHUT, H. *The Restoration of the Self.* New York: Int. Univ. Press, 1977.
24. KOLB, J. E. and GUNDERSON, J. G. "Diagnosing Borderline Patients with a Semi-Structural Interview," *Arch. Gen. Psychiat.*, 37:37-41, 1980.
25. KRYSTAL, H. "Alexithymia and Psychotherapy," *Am. J. Psychotherapy*, 23:17-31, 1979.
26. MACK, J. E. (Ed.). *Borderline States in Psychiatry.* New York: Grune & Stratton, 1975.
27. MAGNAN, V. *Leçons cliniques, 2nd. Edit.*, Paris: Bataille, 1893.
28. MAHLER, M. S. *On Human Symbiosis and the Vicissitudes of Individuation, Vol. 1, Infantile Psychosis.* New York: Int. Univ. Press, 1968.
29. MAHLER, M. S. "A Study of the Separation-Individuation Process and Its Possible Application to Borderline Phenomena in the Psychoanalytic Situation," *The Psychoanalytic Study of the Child*, 26:403-424, 1971.
30. MAHLER, M. S. and FURER, M. "Certain Aspects of the Separation-Individuation Phase," *Psychoanal. Quart.*, 32:1-14, 1963.
31. MANDELL, A. J. "Psychoanalysis and Psychopharmacology" in: Marmor, J. (Ed.), *Modern Psychoanalysis.* New York: Basic Books, 274-290, 1968.
32. MARTY, P. and DE M'UZAN. "La pensée opératoire," *Rev. PsychoAnal.*, (Suppl) 27:1345-1456, 1963.
33. MASTERSON, J. F. "Treatment of the Adolescent with Borderline Syndrome: A Problem in Separation-Individuation," *Bull. Menninger Clinic*, 35:5-18, 1971.

34. MASTERSON, J. F. *Treatment of the Borderline Adolescent: A Developmental Approach.* New York: Wiley, 1972.
35. MASTERSON, J. F. "The Splitting Defence Mechanism of the Borderline Adolescent: Developmental and Clinical Aspects," in: Mack, J. E. (Ed.), *Borderline States in Psychiatry.* New York: Grune & Stratton, 93-102, 1975.
36. MASTERSON, J. F. (Ed). *New Perspectives on Psychotherapy of the Borderline Adult.* New York: Brunner Mazel, 1978.
37. MODELL, A. H. "Primitive Object Relationships and the Predisposition to Schizophrenia," *Internat. J. Psycho-Anal.*, 44:282-292, 1963.
38. NEMIAH, J. C. and SIFNEOS, P. E. "Affect and Fantasy in Psychosomatic Diseases," in Hill, O. W. (Ed.), *Modern Trends in Psychosomatic Medicine, Vol. 2.* London: Butterworth, 26-34.
39. REICH, W. *Character Analysis.* New York: Orgone Press, 1949.
40. SARWER-FONER, G. J. *The Dynamics of Psychiatric Drug Therapy.* Springfield: CC Thomas, 1960.
41. SARWER-FONER, G. J. "A Psychoanalytic Note on a Specific Delusion of Time in Psychotic Depression," *Canad. Psychiat. A. J. Suppl.*, 11:S221-S228, 1966.
42. SARWER-FONER, G. J. "Some Aspects of Anal Object Relationships," *Seminars presented to Students of the Canadian Institute of Psychoanalysis*, 1972-73.
43. SARWER-FONER, G. J. "On Human Territoriality: A Contribution to Instinct Theory," *Canad. Psychiat. A. J. Suppl.*, 17:SS169-183, 1972.
44. SARWER-FONER, G. J. "An Approach to the Global Treatment of the Borderline Patient. Psychoanalytic, Psycho-therapeutic and Psychopharmacolegical Considerations," in: Harticollis, P. (Ed.), *Borderline Conditions.* New York: Int. Univ. Press, 1977.
45. SARWER-FONER, G. J. "Borderline Personality Disorders," in: *Syllabus, Psychiatric Knowledge and Skills Self-Assessment.* Washington, D.C.: Amer. Psychiat. Assoc., 1979.
46. SARWER-FONER, G. J. and KEALEY, L. S. "Reactions to Hospitalization: Passive Dependency Factors, Recurrence of Original Symptoms and Attempts to Prolong Hospitalization on the Announcement of Discharge," *Compreh. Psychiat.*, 22:103-113, 1981.
47. SARWER-FONER, G. J. "On Social Paranoia: The Psychotic Fear of the Stranger and He Who is Alien," *Psychiat. J. Univ. Ottawa*, 4:21-34, 1979.
48. SARWER-FONER, G. J. "Some Thoughts on the Current Status of the Schizophrenic Group of Illnesses: Treatment, Research and Social Aspects," presented at *The 134th Annual Meeting of the American Psychiatric Association*, New Orleans, Louisiana, 1981.
49. SARWER-FONER, G. J. "Denial of Death and the Unconscious Longing for Indestructability and Immortality in the Terminal Phase of Adolescence," *Canad. Psychiat. Assoc. J. Supp.*, 17:SS:51-57, 1972.
50. SIFNEOS, P. E. "The Prevalence of Alexithymic Characteristics in Psy-

chosomatic Patients," *Psychotherapy and Psychosomatics*, Basel: Karger, S., 22:255-262, 1973.
51. SCHMIDEBERG, M. "The Treatment of Psychopathic and Borderline Patients," *Amer. J. Psychother.*, 1:45-70, 1947.
52. SCHMIDEBERG, M. "The Borderline Patient," in: Arieti, S. (Ed.), *American Handbook of Psychiatry*, Vol. 1:398-416, New York: Basic Books, 1959.
53. STENGEL, E. "A Study of Some Clinical Aspects of the Relationship between Obsessional Neurosis and Psychotic Reactions Types," *J. Men. Sci.*, 91:166-187, 1945.
54. STERN, A. "Psychoanalytic Therapy in the Borderline Neuroses," *Psychoanal. Quart.*, 14:190-198, 1945.
55. TARTAKOFF, H. H. et al. "The Normal Personality in Our Culture and the Nobel Prize Complex," in: Loewenstein, R. M., Newman, L. N., Schur, M. and Solnit, A. J. (Eds.), *Psychoanalysis—A General Psychology*. New York: Int. Univ. Press, 222-252, 1966.
56. ZETZEL, E. R. "A Developmental Approach to the Borderline Patient," *Amer. J. Psychiat.*, 127:867-871, 1971.
57. ZILBOORG, G. "Ambulatory Schizophrenias," *Psychiatry*, 4:149-155, 1941.

Chapter 6

The Treatment of the Severe Schizophrenic Patient

Robert Cancro, M.D.

INTRODUCTION

This chapter is written with the clinician in mind. It reflects the clinical experience of the author to a greater degree and the scientific literature to a lesser degree than is usually the case in a published article. There will be a deemphasis on theoretical issues in an effort to highlight those which are of more clinical relevance. The category of schizophrenia has been conceptualized quite differently by different observers. To this day different clinicians mean very different things when they speak of the schizophrenic disorders. It is, therefore, useful to look at how the concept evolved and how it was used in the past before I describe how it will be used in this chapter.

The term was introduced by Morel in 1852 to describe a young patient. This adolescent patient showed impairment of cognitive functioning which Morel described as *demence precoce*. He did not intend to describe an illness, let alone a disease entity. He was merely describing the clinically interesting features of a case of dementia in an adolescent boy. Kraepelin borrowed the term and Latinized it into *dementia praecox*. Kraepelin meant something quite specific and was actually trying to describe a disease entity. In his efforts to create a scientific classification, he separated a large group of mental patients, in whom cognition was impaired in the direction of illogicality, into two groups: those who tended to deteriorate and those who did not. He assumed that these different outcomes neatly divided the patients into two distinct disease entities. The terms dementia praecox and manic-depressive psychosis were meant to describe entities which had different natural courses and outcomes. As naive as this approach may sound, it was a remarkable insight. There are very few concepts in psychiatry that are still in use 85 years after their introduction, let alone have proven to be as valuable as has this distinction.

Eugen Bleuler did not just change the name of the illness but made an important theoretical move away from Kraepelin's position. While Kraepelin was searching for disease entities, Bleuler was creating syndromes. He saw the schizophrenias as a group of illnesses and not as a single disease. He felt these illnesses shared certain features in common, but that they were different disorders having different etiologies, different pathogeneses, different courses and different outcomes. Bleuler also approached his data with a theoretical preconception which he imposed on the observational data. He believed that the basic lesion of this group of disorders had to do with the failure of synthesis of different mental functions—ergo the term schizophrenia. He felt there was a splitting of mental functioning and a loss of the natural harmony of the mind. It is true, nevertheless, that Bleuler was almost as pessimistic as Kraepelin concerning recovery. He defined schizophrenia as a group of illnesses which never permitted full restitution to the premorbid level of personality functioning.

Kraepelin, like Jaspers, tended to look upon the content of psychoses as incomprehensible. The illness was of interest but not the altered communications. Freud deviated importantly from this more Germanic tradition of psychiatry. Freud recognized that psychoses were comprehensible but required a process of decoding the language in which psychotic verbalizations were made. He believed there was order and lawfulness to psychotic symptoms and that they could be understood. Nevertheless, even Freud had in mind, by his use of the term schizophrenia or dementia praecox, patients who tended to require long-term care for their chronic illnesses.

ETIOLOGY

A great deal or very little is known about the etiology of these disorders, depending on your perspective. It is obviously a good deal of information if you have to memorize it, but it is very little if you have the illness. What we know, however, does tell us with clarity that biologic factors are involved at least to a statistically significant degree. That statement does not mean that every patient is biologically loaded. It does not even mean that there are patients who are not biologically loaded. It merely means that our classification of the schizophrenic disorders has a very poor signal-to-noise ratio and that there are many patients included in the group simply because at one moment in time they had certain symptoms. The symptoms used by any currently popular diagnostic scheme will define a group of people who have arrived at the symptoms through very different mechanisms and pathways. The group is not biologically homogenous and, therefore, any study of the biology of the disorder will suffer accordingly. The surprise is that research such as the genetic studies shows statistical significance, rather than that the significance is modest.

This point may be clarified in another way. Family studies reveal that first-degree relatives of schizophrenics, i.e., siblings, parents and offspring, are 10 times as likely to have an illness diagnosed as schizophrenic as are the first-degree relatives of someone not so diagnosed. A tenfold increase in the likelihood of an event is highly impressive. Viewed from another perspective, 90% of the first-degree relatives fail to show a schizophrenic illness, and this is also very impressive. An event which has a probability of 10% can be looked upon as frequent or rare, depending upon the values of the observer. If there is a 10% risk that a plane will crash, this seems quite high to its occupants, but may not be so impressive to those on the ground. The numbers can, in other words, be misleading unless they are placed in perspective. In summary, it can be said that both biologic and nonbiologic factors operate in the etiology of this group of disorders. They operate interactively to produce different predispositions, which are initiated by different factors and evolve along different pathways to produce similar end states. These end states are called schizophrenia, but it should be remembered that the process of arriving at the end state can also be called schizophrenia.

DIAGNOSIS

A heterogeneous syndrome, the diagnosis of which cannot be validated through an independent method, will have different criteria for its diagnosis at different times. These criteria will vary as a function of which diagnostic system is popular at a given moment. Kraepelin's diagnoses were based on the typical case. He described signs and symptoms which were typical, and the clinician was expected to compare the actual patient to a mental template of a typical case and make a diagnostic decision. Obviously, considerable experience and judgement were required.

Bleuler's position was much less empirical. He had a theory of the schizophrenic disorders, and he identified a group of altered fundamental signs which were the basis for diagnosing the group of illnesses. These signs were popular for many years but their use required clinical inferences. The fundamental signs do not readily lend themselves to checklists and, in particular, do not lend themselves to direct patient inquiry. The clinician cannot ask the patient whether or not he is experiencing a loosening of associations.

Langfeldt attempted to reduce this nosologic confusion by separating a core group which he called true schizophrenia from other illnesses, which he called schizophrenic psychoses. He put great emphasis on symptoms such as depersonalization, derealization, estrangement, emotional blunting, and autism. Langfeldt was able to make good prognostic use of this approach but its replication in the hands of other workers has been limited.

Schneider studied a group of patients about whom there was general diagnostic agreement. He identified those symptoms which were present in these patients and differentiated them from other patients about whom there was less diagnostic agreement. He indicated that these were symptoms of the first rank of importance. Schneider did not intend for a clinical judgement to be replaced by a symptom list. It is an unfortunate fact that ideas are often misunderstood and misapplied. Schneider emphasized the importance of clinical judgement and that the search for first-rank symptoms was not a substitute for a careful examination of the patient. It is sad that Schneider's approach has been reduced to a checklist which often eliminates all clinical inference and judgement.

DSM-III is not as empirical as Schneider nor as theoretical as Bleuler. In a very real sense, it is more a political compromise between contending points of view. It emphasizes reliability and deemphasizes clinical inference and/or intuition. It also emphasizes the importance of descriptive approaches and recognizes the need to examine the patient in a multiaxial fashion. In a certain sense it has become too mechanistic and attempts to simulate clinical inference by a decision tree model which does not capture the complexity of clinical judgement.

The bias of this author is to use a modification of Bleuler's criteria and to put great emphasis on the disorganization of the cognitive process traditionally known as thought disorder. This approach requires clinical inference and does not lend itself as neatly to a checklist format.

SYMPTOMS

In speaking of symptom severity it is necessary to make a distinction between severity as the degree of deviation and severity as a prognostic indicator. Symptoms such as hallucinations differ markedly from the usual life experiences. In that sense they are the most severe. Nevertheless they are usually associated with a better prognosis. The more florid the positive symptoms, the more likely is the outcome to be a good one. Symptoms which are much less deviant than delusions and hallucinations carry much more grave prognoses. These include anhedonia, apathy, anergia, and withdrawal. These so-called negative symptoms, while not as dramatic, are much more likely to be associated with a poor outcome.

It is probably best to use outcome or resistance to treatment as the best indicator of severity. However psychotic a person may appear at a moment in time, if he recovers and does well the illness is not as severe as one which results in long-term disability. Prognosis then becomes the equivalent of severity. Unfortunately, much more is known about the factors which are predictive of outcome than those which are determinants of it. The younger the age of onset of the illness, the worse the prognosis. This may be because early-onset schizophrenic psychoses are the more malignant types or because of a diminished differentiation of the personality at the time of onset of the illness. In general, a paranoid schizophrenic disorder carries a better prognosis than a nonparanoid one. It is not clear why this is true. Similarly, good premorbid social adjustment is predictive of good outcome, but the reasons are uncertain. The presence of depression as part of the acute psychotic decompensation carries a good prognosis.

INTRODUCTION TO TREATMENT

There are some general points about the treatment of schizophrenic patients which are worth making as an introduction to the topic. An important variable is the attitude of the therapist to the patient. To some degree all of the contributors to this volume have been advocates for particular groups of people. All advocates have a tendency to believe that the group they advocate has suffered the most. As in all paranoid positions there is a tendency to be convinced that everyone else is wrong. There are some data, however, to support the position that schizophrenics have been served poorly. Very few communities will accept large numbers of schizophrenic patients. If elderly patients are discharged into a community there will be grumbling, but if schizophrenic patients are discharged into that same community there will be an uproar. It is rationalized in many ways, not the least of which is that the patients set a poor example for the children, but it is clear that madness in this form is not accepted by the population readily.

The study of the history of the treatment of schizophrenia shows that these patients have been brutalized for as long as we have written records. In the name of help, harm has been done with regularity. Terror and intimidation were seen as important treatment techniques. It was emphasized into the early 19th century that fear was an important treatment modality for chronic madness. Fear was conceived as a method of shocking people back into rationality. A variety of techniques were used, including immersing people in wells, throwing people from great heights into bodies of water, and submerging people under water in coffin-like boxes until air bubbles ceased to rise.

Around the time of World War I we moved into a more quasiscientific approach to madness. At this time we saw the use of intrathecal horse serum, the administration of gold salts and the treatment of focal infections. Hospitals were crowded with edentulous patients whose teeth had been removed to treat the focal infections whose existence had never been demonstrated. The surgeons were not far behind the dentists with their hemithyroidectomies, gonadectomies and other mutilating procedures. As late as the 1950's psychosurgical techniques were used which involved the random and uncontrolled destruction of nervous tissue in the name of therapy. There is a long history of destructive intervention rationalized as being for the benefit of the patient. It is generous to conclude that these interventions reflect ambivalence and not unalloyed sadism. The chronic schizophrenic has the capacity to elicit intense negative feelings. The professional not uncommonly reacts to these negative feelings with a so-called therapeutic fervor which quickly crosses into excessive zeal. It is not always clear when "doing something for them" shades imperceptibly into "doing something to them."

It is always essential to keep in mind the therapeutic goals of the intervention. Therapeutic goals may be quite restrictive and include only psychotic symptom amelioration. Given this definition, when the person no longer hallucinates he has recovered, independent of the quality of the adjustment. Such a person may be withdrawn and may not lead a productive life but still be considered symptomatically improved. Other colleagues define improvement in more psychodynamic terms and strive for some absolute standard of mental health. Others put much more emphasis on social and vocational functioning. The best general definition of improvement borrows from all three of these approaches to include measures of quality of life, personality growth and differentiation, and freedom from psychotic symptoms.

The very heterogeneity of the etiopathogeneses described earlier means that the disorder comes about in different ways in different people. There must, therefore, be a range of therapeutic interventions which matches the diversity of etiopathogeneses. There can be no single nor even a preferred treatment for people who differ in every meaningful parameter of the illness except some symptoms which have been endowed with diagnostic importance. There must be a range of treatment modalities available. The fact that a person is responsive to a particular treatment does not necessarily shed light on the origin of the illness. Someone may respond to psychosocial intervention without that indicating the psychosocial sphere is the origin of the illness. Conversely, a response to a somatic treatment does not mean that somatic factors must have been involved in initiating the disorder. The pain that complicates a terminal cancer may respond to social contact but this does not mean that the pain is psychosocial in origin. Similarly, the day-to-day anxieties of life may respond to alcohol or social drugs without verifying that these anxieties derived from the biology of the person. The identification of useful treatments is empirical. Their utility does not necessarily shed light on etiology or on pathogenesis.

PSYCHOPHARMACOLOGY

If there is anything close to a standard treatment of the schizophrenic disorders, it is psychopharmacologic treatment. Unfortunately, drugs have become the treatment of choice for almost everyone and everything to some degree. The amount of anxiolytic medication consumed by the American population is frightening. This misuse only serves to illustrate how convenient drugs can be as an alternative to a more comprehensive effort. The misuse of psychopharmacology should not serve as an excuse for its abandonment. Psychopharmacologic drugs are useful and have made a major contribution to the treatment of the schizophrenic disorders. The drugs have not cured a schizophrenic. The recovery rates for schizophrenia have not changed particularly in the last 80 years. There is no increase in the percentage of people recovering. The drugs have made a major contribution, however, in hastening the tempo of recovery and keeping people out of hospitals. The psychopharmacologic agents have been particularly useful for acute schizophrenia. They are helpful in the chronic disorders, but to a lesser degree. They have not been particularly helpful for the negative symptoms of anhedonia, social withdrawal, anergia, apathy, listlessness, indifference, etc. Psychosocial treatments seem to be more useful for the negative symptoms.

Clinicians should try to master a handful of drugs and not attempt to become familiar with all of them. The in-depth understanding of a few drugs is to be preferred over a superficial familiarity with many drugs. The clinician must always weigh the costs and the benefits of any treatment. There has recently been considerable emphasis on the risk of tardive dyskinesia, but this is only one of the problems in the use of medication. Any treatment which is efficacious is also dangerous. The drugs should be used intelligently, carefully and with respect. There should be specific target symptoms, and these target symptoms should be ones which are likely to be responsive to medication. Antipsychotic agents should not be used as hypnotics nor as anxiolytics. There is no clinician known to this author who prescribes chlorpromazine to family members who "want a good night's sleep." It is an excellent rule of thumb that if it is not good enough for your family, it is not good enough for your patients.

INDIVIDUAL PSYCHOTHERAPY

During the psychopharmacologic era the role of individual psychotherapy has diminished sharply. There have been studies which have failed to demonstrate the utility of psychotherapy, and this negative finding has been interpreted incorrectly by many people as a positive demonstration of ineffectiveness. It has been repeatedly demonstrated that some patients respond to individual psychotherapy. This is not surprising when one realizes that all human beings are social creatures who can be influenced by other human beings. Being schizophrenic does not make one oblivious to this kind of interpersonal pressure. It is very common, for example, to see rapid and dramatic changes in an individual who falls in love. Many features of the loved one are incorporated into the individual's personality. This is not to suggest that schizophrenic patients should fall in love with their therapists; it merely illustrates that intense involvement with another human being can have a dramatic and important impact on people. The schizophrenic disorders make it more difficult to relate, but they do not prevent the patient from developing an intense relationship.

It is more difficult to develop a relationship with a schizophrenic patient because, as a rule, these patients are masters at creating uncertainty and ambiguity. The therapist does not usually accept these qualities comfortably. The neurotic patient, unlike the schizophrenic, tends to demonstrate the positive transference openly and clearly. The neurotic patient tends to invest the therapist with remarkable powers and qualities. The schizophrenic patient does not indulge in this particular set of fantasies. The schizophrenic, if anything, seems more aware of the therapist's unconscious than the therapist may like. Often the patient is rejecting and superficially negative towards the therapist. This lack of positive reinforcement can cause the therapist to withdraw and lose interest.

Work with these patients requires considerable flexibility. They are not always willing to be seen from exactly 9:00 to 9:45. They may come to the office at times when they have not been scheduled or not come at times when they have appointments. They may not wish to leave at the end of what the therapist feels is a reasonable period of time. All of these behaviors can be disconcerting and disruptive. It is essential that the therapist be willing to adapt to the peculiar needs of such people if the treatment is to offer any assistance.

Individual psychotherapy with these patients requires a resoluteness, perhaps even a stubbornness, on the part of the therapist. The therapist must be able to make a commitment to such a patient and to remain steadfast to that commitment for a long period of time despite severe testing. These patients tend to be very sensitive to whether you are being truthful with them or whether you are behaving in a less than honest fashion. They will assess your trustworthiness in a variety of ways which at times border on the ingenious. It is almost necessary to fail some of the tests before the patient can assess you adequately. When a therapist fails to recognize a trap, falls into it, and still behaves in a reasonable and decent fashion, it says a great deal about the therapist as a person. How the therapist handles these blows is very informative to the patient.

OTHER TREATMENTS

There are a variety of group, family and social support interventions which can be enormously helpful to such patients. Family attitudes including rejection, criticism, and hostility play a critical role in the relapse rate, at least in certain patients. The ability of the family to tolerate and accept the patient can prevent rehospitalization. As is always the case in working with schizophrenia, there is the problem of finding the channel between Scylla and Charybdis. If the family is not sufficiently involved, the patient may regress, but if the family is too involved, the patient may decompensate. Family treatment can be particularly helpful in determining the right balance.

Alternatives to hospitalization such as Soteria House are useful for certain kinds of patients, particularly in terms of the quality of their social outcome. These alternative modes of treatment can be less expensive than traditional methods. Nevertheless, it is necessary to recognize that no matter what therapeutic modality is utilized, a significant percentage of these patients are going to show social and vocational deficits. These deficits may respond in part to rehabilitative techniques. Vocational deficits have been overcome in a number of countries which have placed emphasis on rehabilitation. The cost of schizophrenia to the gross national product of the United States has been estimated at between 15 and 20 billion dollars. The major part of this cost is a consequence of underemployment. The investment in rehabilitation is very likely to be economically fruitful. There is no adequate measure of the social cost borne by these people and their families.

The personal relationship between the physician and the patient is essential in the treatment of any patient, including a schizophrenic. You cannot treat schizophrenia any more successfully than you can treat diabetes without a strong doctor/patient relationship. A key feature in this relationship is a measure of optimism and hope on the part of the physician. The vast majority of these patients ultimately do tend to go into remission if only they live long enough. The clinician serves a critical role in trying to sustain life so that this person can live to the point where he is likely to go into a more complete remission. It is difficult to develop a strong doctor/patient relationship in the face of the communications deficit which characterizes these patients. It is perhaps only the experience and sense of mutual trust that can develop in an intense dyadic relationship which can bridge this gap.

SUGGESTED READINGS

1. BLEULER, E. *Dementia Praecox, or the Group of the Schizophrenias.* New York: IUP, 1950.
2. CANCRO, R. "Overview of Schizophrenia," in: Kaplan, H. I., Freedman, A. M. and Sadock, B. J. (Eds.), *Comprehensive Textbook of Psychiatry/III.* Baltimore: Williams & Wilkins, 1980.
3. GOTTESMAN, I. I. and SHIELDS, J. "A Critical Review of Recent Adoption, Twin, and Family Studies of Schizophrenia: Behavioral Genetics Perspectives," *Schizophr. Bull.* 2:360, 1976.
4. LANGFELDT, G. "The Prognosis in Schizophrenia," *Acta Psychiatr. Scand. (Suppl)* 110:1, 1956.
5. LIDZ, T., FLECK, S. and CORNELISON, A. *Schizophrenia & the Family.* New York: IUP, 1965.
6. SCHNEIDER, K. *Clinical Psychopathology.* New York: Grune & Stratton, 1959.

Index